MARK MAHANEY

KUNDALINI
YOGA

UNLOCK
YOUR INNER
POTENTIAL
THROUGH
LIFE-CHANGING
EXERCISE

BY SHAKTA KAUR KHALSA

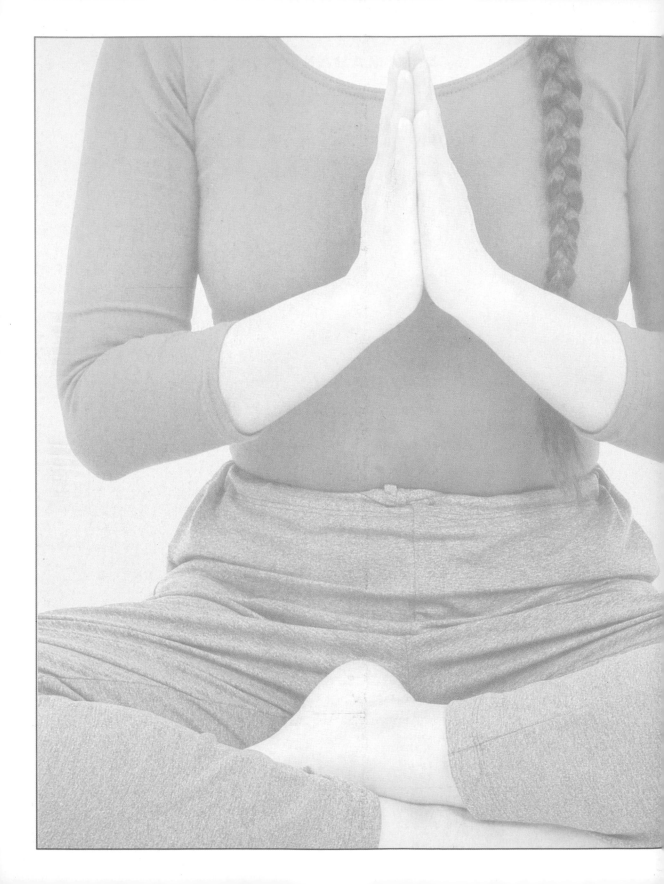

KUNDALINI
YOGA

AS TAUGHT BY YOGI BHAJAN

UNLOCK
YOUR INNER
POTENTIAL
THROUGH
LIFE-CHANGING
EXERCISE

BY SHAKTA KAUR KHALSA

APPROVED BY THE
KUNDALINI RESEARCH INSTITUTE

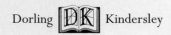

Dorling **DK** Kindersley

LONDON, NEW YORK, SYDNEY, DEHLI,
PARIS, MUNICH, AND JOHANNESBURG

Project Editors Barbara M. Berger and Crystal A. Coble
Book Designer Mandy Earey
DTP Designer Jill Bunyan
Production Manager David Proffit
Category Publisher LaVonne Carlson
Art Director Tina Vaughan
Cover Art Director Dirk Kaufman
Photographer Dave King
Editorial Consultant KRI Institute

First American Edition, 2001
01 02 03 04 05 10 9 8 7 6 5 4 3

Published in the United States by
Dorling Kindersley Publishing, Inc.
95 Madison Avenue
New York, New York 10016

DK Publishing offers special discounts for bulk purchases for sales
promotions or premiums. Specific, large-quantity needs can be met with
special editions, including personalized covers, excerpts of existing guides,
and corporate imprints. For more information, contact Special Markets
Department, DK Publishing, Inc., 95 Madison Avenue, New York, NY 10016
Fax: 800-600-9098.

Cataloging in Publication data is available from the Library of Congress
ISBN 0-7894-6770-4

Color reproduction by Colourscan, Singapore
Printed and bound in China by L.Rex Printing Co. Ltd.

See our complete catalog at
www.dk.com

CONTENTS

FOREWORD

Shakta Kaur Khalsa has given us a place to start. Every journey needs a good first step—firm and well-placed—and the right direction to find the path to your chosen destination. This book helps the beginner with that first step. And for those with prior experience in Kundalini Yoga, this book will become a treasure of information and inspiration.

Shakta answers the questions that remove any initial hesitation to try Kundalini Yoga, even if it is something completely new to you: What is its nature? Where did it come from? How will it benefit me? Is it dangerous? Can I do what I do in the world and still do this?

She goes even further to give us the answers we need to feel confident and actually try these techniques: What do I need to know to begin? What exercises do I do first? What things can I try for specific physical and mental benefits? How do I design and develop my own practice? How does this apply to my daily life to make it a little better? Her descriptions and fine graphics set a clear path to explore these exercises and meditations.

Why produce such a book now? There are many books on yoga and exercise. After reading this book, I decided there are four main reasons for her to write this and for us to read this particular book:

1 **The use of yoga exercise and meditation** has moved from an interest only for specialists and people at society's fringe in the early 1960s to the mainstream in the new millennium. Thousands of research investigations have proven its usefulness for health, mental clarity and a sense of spirit. Everyone does it from executives to sports teams to the average person trying to drop a few pounds and take a deep breath to conquer stress.

2 **With increased awareness and interest** in the many benefits of yoga, it has become the practice of families and of "householders"- people involved in the usual challenges at work and in families. Many traditions of yoga began with a focus on people who removed themselves from normal life. They were monks, celibates, seekers, renunciates, and even hermits. They felt spirit was in some way removed from the domain of a working life and needed to be cultivated away from the distractions and temptations we face each day. Kundalini yoga was the exception. It had and has an attitude distinct from this. It was practiced and designed for people who wanted to be healthy, happy, and holy while fully in the world—working, tending families, serving in the armies, running organizations, and even participating in politics. It was designed to be fast and powerful to give you the strength and integrity to master your mind and deliver your values with integrity in your life. So the spread of yoga to everyone in every walk of life has brought the techniques of Kundalini Yoga to center stage.

3 **The demands on each of us** in this globalized, fast-paced, connected world of information and change must be balanced with a renewed awakening of spirit. Without a strong sense of spirit we can become overwhelmed by the very wealth of choices we have created and the number of relationships we are in. We need a way to become still, listen to our heart, and know who we are and why we make the choices we do. Kundalini Yoga and meditation are perfect tools for this. With them we can open our senses, identify our conflicts, and call on our intelligence and our intuition to go beyond our conflicts.

4 **Shakta Kaur** is a good writer and educator. She has delighted adults and children with her books characterized by ease of use, artistic design, and accuracy of information.

Put all these together and you probably want to skip the rest of this introduction and leap into her exposition. So, I will conclude quickly with one last observation.

As the director of training and certification for Kundalini yoga in the Kundalini Research Institute and in 3HO International for almost 30 years, I have seen the power the practice of Kundalini yoga has to transform the lives of individuals. Put aside wild claims you may have heard. I will tell you what really happens.

With a regular practice you remember you are a human being. You are not a thing. Your are not just animal. Neither are you some angel. You are a human being first. You have the power to commit, to speak your heart in words, to open your mind to vastness across time and space, and to love without limit. Yoga helps you do just that.

Where you have held back, you begin to move ahead. You create an exceptional life and embrace it with gratitude. You realize life can be lived unconsciously or consciously and you choose awareness. You tap new energy and resources within yourself. You develop a meditative mind that can sense the impact of your decisions before you make them. You develop a presence and even become enlightened. Yogi Bhajan, the master teacher who shared all of this with us, was asked what it means to be enlightened. He responded: "You have the capacity and the habit to speak words without darkness. You rely on your grace as your essential power." Someone then asked, "What does it mean to have grace?" He said, "You have the practice of meditative innocence." Yoga ultimately gives you yourself with inner trust and self-dignity.

Kundalini Yoga does not make you levitate above the ground. It does give you the ability to elevate your mind and your life. It does not turn you into a gymnast. It does give you flexibility for a normal life. It does not remove you or block you from deep involvement in all aspects of social, professional and family life. It does help you remove the common blocks to a fulfilled life.

With this book as a good first step, I know the rest of your journey will be exciting, fruitful, and full of awareness.

—*Gurucharan Singh Khalsa, Ph.D.,* co-author of *Breathwalk* and *The Mind* with *Yogi Bhajan, Ph.D.,* director of training for Kundalini Yoga and KRI

INTRODUCTION
ROOTS OF YOGA

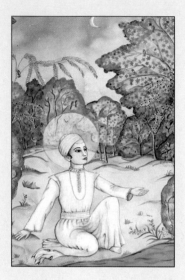

Thousands of years ago, highly evolved humans created the system of yoga. The science of the care, maintenance, and preservation of the human body, mind, and spirit was guarded through the centuries.

"A majority of the people who like to live peaceful, tranquil lives with strength and compassion, with character and commitment, will come to yoga and practice whichever form of yoga their good luck brings them."

–Yogi Bhajan

The word yoga comes from the ancient Indian language called Sanskrit, and it means union. It can be thought of as a yoke, of sorts, binding together the body, mind, and spirit. Ultimately, yoga is the union of the individual's unit consciousness with the infinite consciousness. Although it can be practiced religiously each day, yoga is not a religion. A more accurate description of yoga would be to say that it is an ancient science.

Early forms of yoga were formulated as long as 10,000 years ago. Some of the oldest records of yoga were found in scrolls from ancient Tibet. As a universally known technology for raising consciousness, yoga has its roots in many ancient cultures, such as the Chinese, Indian, and Mayan. Of these, Indian culture has been the most well-known source, and the treasure keeper of yoga for thousands of years. Evidence of the concept and practice of meditation was found in the excavated remains of two ancient cities in India, which dated back before 1800 B.C. As centuries went by, cave- and forest-dwelling yogis guarded this sacred science. The science of the care, maintenance and preservation of the human body, mind, and spirit was guarded through the centuries, and passed on from individual masters to select students who were deemed worthy.

During the Classical Epoch (A.D. 200-800), the technologies of yoga were systematized. Eventually a portion of this vast knowledge was recorded and preserved. Out of the classical period of yoga philosophy emerged a prominent codification of yoga, the Patanjali Sutras, which are still considered the foundation of yoga today. In brief, the eight-fold path described therein is as follows: Yama (the five restraints, such as nonviolence, sensory control), Nivama (the five disciplines, such as surrender, purity), Asana (postures for health), Pranayama (control of breath), Pratyhara (synchronization of senses and thoughts), Dharana (one-pointed concentration), Dhyana (deep meditation), and Samadhi (awakening and absorption in spirit).

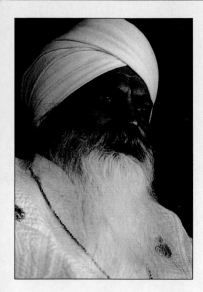

Yogi Bhajan
Master of Kundalini Yoga
Founder of 3HO

Classical yoga includes the well-known Hatha Yoga, which generally has emphasis on Asana, or postures. The purpose of Hatha Yoga is to raise the consciousness. Toward this end, Kundalini Yoga and Hatha Yoga are the same, as all rivers ultimately flow to the sea. The difference is how long it takes to get there, and what is experienced along the way. Originally Classical Yoga was intended for monks, yogis, and those who withdrew from the world for spiritual practice. Kundalini Yoga, on the other hand, was designed for the householder, those who live in the world, who have families and jobs, and who want to balance the inner and outer world. It is the yoga that fits the busy lives most of us lead. Kundalini Yoga, which includes many asanas found in Hatha Yoga, is effective, efficient, and easy. Those who practice it say they can feel changes in the body and psyche within a few minutes, and deeper changes through regular practice.

The process of yoga focuses on the need to control the "waves" of the mind. The mind is considered to be the link between the body and the spirit, or consciousness. The habits of the mind can bind us to the temporal life—called maya, or "illusion"—which, by its very nature, consists of pairs of opposites (happy/sad, good/bad). On the other hand, this very same mind leads us to merge with the Infinite.

The yoga described in these pages is but a sampling of the vast wealth of Kundalini Yoga, based on the teachings of Yogi Bhajan, Ph.D. Kundalini Yoga was never taught publicly, until Yogi Bhajan challenged the age-old tradition of secrecy. In 1969, in his compassionate wisdom, Yogi Bhajan brought Kundalini Yoga to the United States, from which it has spread all over the world. His reasoning, given in his own words, is as follows: "I am sharing these teachings to create a science of the total self . . . It is the birthright of every human being to be healthy, happy, and holy." The master of Kundalini Yoga, and head of the Sikh faith for the Western Hemisphere, Yogi Bhajan is also the founder of 3HO (Healthy, Happy, Holy Organization), a worldwide non-profit foundation which offers classes in Kundalini Yoga, meditation, vegetarian nutrition, and healthy life choices.

Kundalini comes from the word kundal, which means "lock of hair from the beloved." The uncoiling of this "hair" is the awakening of the kundalini, the creative potential that already exists in every human.

This book is intended as a complement to instruction from trained Kundalini Yoga teachers. Personal guidance from a trained teacher, and the experience of group yoga classes are just as important as the guidance from this book. See the Resources section to locate qualified instructors in your area.

THE MYTHS OF KUNDALINI

The myth that kundalini is dangerous could only be possible through extreme mispractice of the technology of kundalini. That is why the practice of Kundalini Yoga, as given by a master of Kundalini Yoga, is essential. Proper technique and preparation is the insulation needed for the proper flow of kundalini energy.

Sometimes the talk of fear and danger can become the biggest danger. In reality, there is the universal spirit, sometimes referred to as God. God uncoils him/her/itself. This uncoiling process is known as kundalini. What is uncoiling is you, nothing more and nothing less. It is a normal capacity that most people simply are not utilizing. If you start utilizing that energy, where is the danger?

Another myth is that a teacher will "initiate" the kundalini in his student. The kundalini can be stimulated directly by a teacher, but toward what end? Just to give an experience that will not be maintained? The gradual awakening process, stimulated by the practitioner's own efforts, activates the flow of kundalini energy in a natural progression.

Some think that to have a kundalini experience means you have gone into a deep trance and are "beyond this world." On the contrary, raising the kundalini energy integrates you more fully with reality, and gives you awareness so that you can act more effectively in higher consciousness.

The King of the Yogis

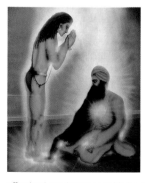

From the chronicles of old India comes the story of a yogi who was considered by all as the king of the yogis. His name was Baba Siri Chand. He had lived for generations, yet looked as youthful as a young man. He had spent his life in samadhi, merged in the blissful absorption of the Infinite One, so his body had not aged. He could perform miracles effortlessly, and transport his body wherever he wanted. He was held in such awe as the king of yogis that even his name was not spoken lightly. It came about that a saintly man named Ram Das was given the title of Guru, which literally means "that which takes you from darkness (gu) to light (ru)." Guru Ram Das was the fourth of the Sikh Gurus, and known for his humility, love, and service to humankind. Upon hearing of the appointment, Baba Siri Chand was much bothered. He felt certain that he should be the Guru—after all, he was the greatest yogi that had ever lived! He could do anything he wanted. All of creation would come and serve him at his command. With these thoughts in mind, he decided to pay the Guru a visit. Guru Ram Das was sitting in meditation as an angry and indignant Baba Siri Chand approached. As he came close, Guru Ram Das opened his eyes and smiled at him with a gracious and kind welcome. Guru Ram Das then took hold of his long beard, and began to brush the dust from the feet of Baba Siri Chand. At this, Baba Siri Chand was speechless. Immediately he understood why Ram Das was the true Guru and not himself. He bowed to Guru Ram Das, saying, "On you I bestow the title of king of the yogis, for you have shown that the true yogi is the selfless servant of the Divine in all."

HOW
IT WORKS

In the physical body, the kundalini resides in the spine. The two nerve channels that intertwine around the central nerve of the spinal column are called the Ida (the lunar, negative energy) and the Pingala (the solar, positive energy). Each of them makes two and one-half turns around the central column of the spine, called the shushmana, as they spiral upward from the base of the spine. The two channels act as main conductors of the kundalini energy, feeding the entire nervous system. Beside the kundalini energy that is already flowing within our bodies, there is a vast reservoir of untapped kundalini stored under the fourth vertebra of the spinal column.

Through the practice of Kundalini Yoga, this untapped energy is stimulated and allowed to rise up the central column of the spine until it reaches the top of the skull, activating the secretion of the pineal gland. This tiny gland (about the size of a grain of wheat in most people) and its function have long been a mystery to Western science. The yogis have known its importance for thousands of years. One of the major functions of the pineal gland is to vibrate and control the nucleus projection of every cell of the body.

All biological consciousness is chemical in nature—it is controlled by the secretion of chemicals in the brain. When we directly raise the kundalini, it causes the activation of these chemicals, and a major change in consciousness is experienced. It may be subtle and gradual. It may be spectacular. Through the consistent practice of Kundalini Yoga, change happens.

This is a yoga for everyday life, and every person. You are not required to be in perfect physical shape or believe anything in particular. Kundalini Yoga works for you if you can breathe and move your body. The gift of Kundalini Yoga is that you experience it. No words can replace that experience. Your experience goes right to your heart, your core. These ancient teachings are designed to give you "hands on" experience of your highest consciousness. By approaching Kundalini Yoga with openness and respect, and by following the steps included in this book, you can change your life.

CHAPTER 1

STARTING AT
GROUND
ZERO

"When the time is on you, start,
and the pressure will be off."
–*Yogi Bhajan*

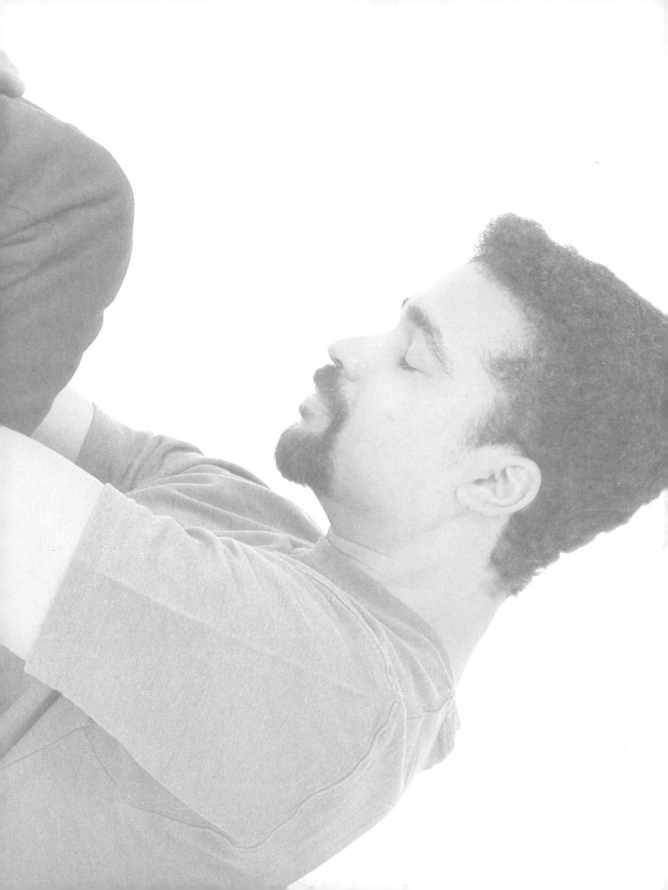

PREPARING YOURSELF

YOUR ENVIRONMENT

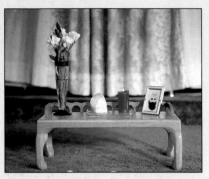

Your Yoga Room Choose a quiet, out-of-the-way space. Add some simple, meaningful decorations and photos on a small altar with a candle. If possible, reserve this space just for yoga and meditation. The room should have a fresh feeling and a moderate temperature. The floor should be padded with carpet; or use a comfortable, thick mat that will not slip.

Your Yoga Mat If you practice yoga on a hard surface, such as a wood floor, be sure to cushion it with a thick pad or blanket. Additionally, a mat of natural fibers such as cotton, wool, silk, or animal skin is recommended for insulation and padding. Wool and sheepskin insulate your electromagnetic field from the earth's energy field. This protects you from becoming tired or drained of energy as you meditate. A pillow placed under the buttocks will help straighten the spine for meditation

Your Yoga Shawl A light, natural fabric shawl or blanket is suggested for meditation and deep relaxation. In meditation, cover the shoulders and spine. If this feels too warm, cover the lower spine only by wrapping the shawl around the waist and lower torso. You should stay comfortably warm during meditation. The body will naturally cool off during the deep relaxation following a yoga set. Covering yourself from the neck down keeps your body temperature constant.

Clothing For yoga, it is best to wear comfortable, elastic-waisted clothing made from a natural fabric, such as cotton. If possible do not wear socks. Bare feet conduct the electromagnetic energy through the 72,000 nerve endings in the feet. Covering the head with a natural fiber cloth, preferably cotton, also strengthens the electromagnetic energy field, and enhances the meditative mind.

Wearing white is preferred, as it is the "infinite" of all colors and is psychologically uplifting.

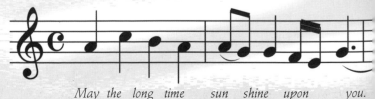

May the long time sun shine upon you.

ADDITIONAL THINGS TO CONSIDER

- Always begin each session by tuning in (see "Before Beginning, Tune In," on page 44).
- Wait at least 1 or, preferably, 2 hours after eating to begin. Empty the bladder before doing yoga.
- Start with the minimum time suggested for an exercise and increase gradually up to the maximum time, but not beyond.
- After choosing a particular yoga set, or kriya, follow it in the order given.
- Generally, a beginning practitioner of Kundalini Yoga will do 30 to 45 minutes of yoga, followed by a 10-minute deep relaxation, and then an 11-minute meditation.
- Drink water after your practice to balance and ground yourself.
- Unless another mantra is given, use *Sat Nam* on the breath.
- Unless specified otherwise, the breathing pattern to use while moving the body is to inhale during expansive, opening movements, and exhale during movements that contract the body. For example, in a forward stretch, inhale while sitting up and exhale while stretching toward your legs.
- Close your eyes and breathe through your nose during yoga, unless instructed otherwise.
- When music is indicated in a yoga set, for relaxation or meditation, it is recommended that you use 3HO music, which is vibrationally compatible with Kundalini Yoga. Hundreds of selections can be ordered from the organizations listed in "Resources".
- **For Women Only:** During the heaviest part of your monthly menses and after the third month of pregnancy, avoid strenuous yoga. In particular do not do the following poses: Bow, Camel, Locust, Root Lock, Shoulder Stand, Plow, Strenuous Leg Lifts, or Breath of Fire.

A Kundalini Yoga class will always end with a special blessing song. To sing along, see the "Resources" section for information on ordering the companion CD especially designed for use with this book. Otherwise you can recite it as an ending poem or blessing. The words are:

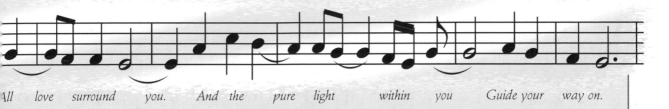

All love surround you. And the pure light within you Guide your way on.

FOCUSING

An important component of Kundalini Yoga and meditation is mental focus. It deepens your awareness of the present moment. After beginning a steady practice, you may find that this becomes an invaluable tool for centering in everyday life.

FOCUS ON THE THIRD-EYE POINT

The mental focus in Kundalini Yoga, unless specified otherwise, is to fix the concentration on the "third-eye point," a point midway between the brows, one-half-inch above the eyebrows and one-half-inch beneath the skin. You can mentally locate this point by closing your eyes and turning them gently upwards and inwards. With practice, you will be able to center your awareness at the third-eye point without the aid of your eyes.

Concentrating on the third-eye point is not intended to block out all other awareness. Remain aware of your breath, your body posture, your movements, and any mantra (mind-guiding sound) you may be using as you center yourself at the third-eye point.

FOCUS WITH A MANTRA

Another aspect of Kundalini Yoga practice that is frequently unspecified is the use of mantra on the breath. Linking a sound with the breath adds to the power of the mental focus.

The mantra most commonly used is *Sat Nam* (rhymes with "But Mom"). *Sat Nam* means "truth is my identity," or "Truth-Identity." This mantra can be linked with the breath by mentally repeating *Sat* as you inhale, and *Nam* as you exhale. By doing so, you connect each thought to a positive outcome.

You will find that the use of a mantra makes it easier to keep up in the practice of any exercise that is particularly strenuous, and that it adds depth to the practice of even the simplest exercise.

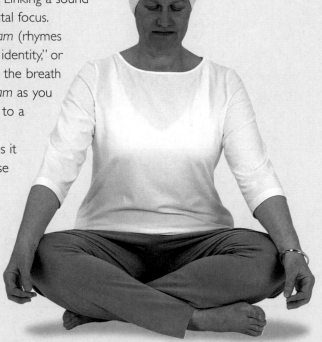

PACING YOURSELF

Many Kundalini kriyas (yoga sets) involve rhythmical movement between two or more postures. Sometimes the pace at which you should move is not stated. As a rule, begin slowly, keeping a steady rhythm. Increase gradually, being careful not to strain. Generally, the more you practice an exercise the faster you can go. In any case, be sure that the spine has become warm and flexible before attempting rapid or strenuous movements.

CONCLUDING AN EXERCISE

Unless otherwise stated, an exercise is concluded by inhaling and holding the breath briefly, then exhaling and relaxing the posture. Keep a strong mental focus, and circulate the energy through the body and mind while holding the breath. Applying the Root Lock on the held inhale is also an option (see page 35 for a discussion of the Root Lock position). This helps to consolidate the effects of the exercise and to circulate energy to the higher centers of the body.

Beginners may hold the breath for 5 to 8 seconds at the conclusion of an exercise. More experienced practitioners may hold the breath longer. In no case, however, should the breath be held to the point of dizziness or faintness. If you begin to experience either, exhale immediately and relax the breath.

RELAXING BETWEEN EXERCISES

The relaxation following an exercise consolidates the effects of that exercise. For this reason, it is important to allow yourself at least a few relaxing breaths between exercises. Ideally, allow for 1 minute of relaxation. Longer periods of relaxation (up to 3 minutes) may be necessary for beginners or for strenuous exercises. Relax in a comfortable position. Unless specified, come into the resting position that is most natural for each exercise. Generally, Easy Pose, Rock Pose, Corpse Pose, or on your stomach (with head turned to the side) are the most common resting poses. Some poses have a natural resting pose that relaxes the body in the opposite stretch. Breathe deeply and consciously. Relax completely with the intention to continue your yoga set. Most kriyas end with a deep relaxation on the back for 10 minutes or more.

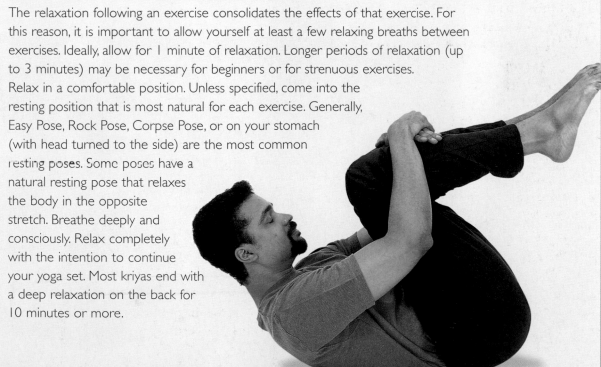

USING
PROPS

Although Kundalini Yoga does not rely on the use of props, as do some other forms of yoga, there are times when the use of props is beneficial. Props can be especially helpful for beginners and anyone who has parts of their body that have not been stretched or exercised for a long time.

Most props, with the exception of the body ball, are common items around the home: a cloth belt or rope, a bolster pillow (from a couch) or thick blankets, a wall, a metal folding chair, a stable desk. Here are some ways these items can help you do yoga.

1 **When muscles** are too tight or weak to hold a posture, backbend on a large ball, bolster pillows, or blankets to open the upper spine. This is especially recommended as preparation for Wheel Pose.

2 **To help** make sitting on the floor more comfortable, place thick blankets, a towel, or a pillow under buttocks to straighten the spine and relax the hips downward. For shoulder stand and plow pose, add a thick blanket under the shoulders and upper back to relieve pressure from the neck.

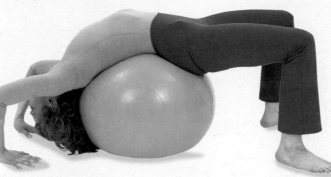

3 **Increase comfort** during relaxation by lying on a rug or mat and placing a rolled up towel or pillow under the knees. This will take pressure off the lower spine. A small, rolled pillow may also be inserted under the neck.

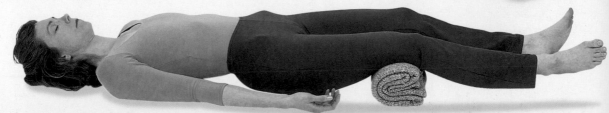

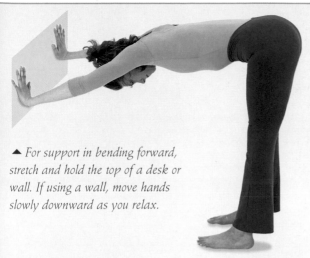

▲ For support in bending forward, stretch and hold the top of a desk or wall. If using a wall, move hands slowly downward as you relax.

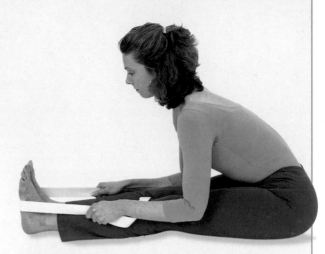

4 For lowering legs in Plow Pose, touch feet to a wall and slowly walk them down toward the floor. Some people find performing Tree Pose easier when standing either with the shoulder and supporting leg next to a wall for support, or with the backs of heels against a wall.

5 To stretch toward the feet, or to grasp arms behind the back, use a strap or rope to cover the distance past where your arms can stretch.

6 For those who cannot sit on the floor to meditate with a straight spine, a chair is an alternative. Use a sturdy, armless, firm-support chair. Place a thick, firm pad or blanket on the chair for sitting on, and a folded blanket under the feet if they are not flat on the ground. Your spine should be straight and lightly supported by the back of the chair.

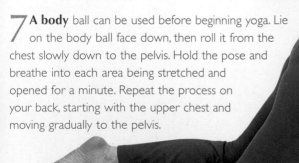

◀ Many exercises, such as Spine Flex and other upper-body exercises, can be performed in a chair. For a good stretch, reach forward with your arms crossed at the forearms.

7 A body ball can be used before beginning yoga. Lie on the body ball face down, then roll it from the chest slowly down to the pelvis. Hold the pose and breathe into each area being stretched and opened for a minute. Repeat the process on your back, starting with the upper chest and moving gradually to the pelvis.

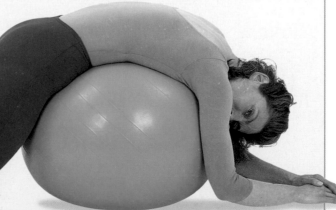

CHAPTER 2

BASICS OF KUNDALINI YOGA

"In me I have found only one reality; that I breathe in and I breathe out. And so anything that breathes in or out is reality. When I found this as a reality in everybody, I found myself in everybody and everybody in myself."

–*Yogi Bhajan*

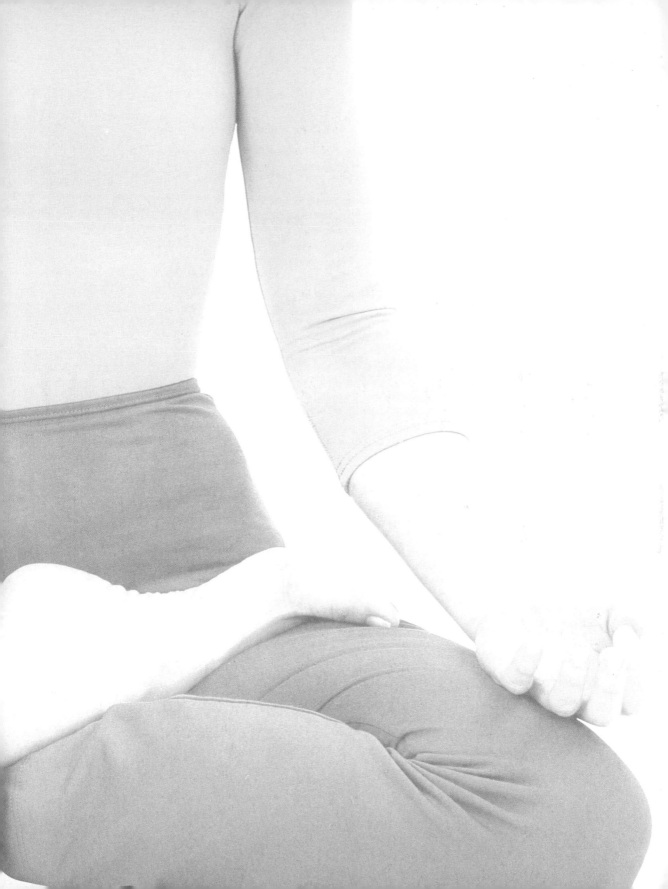

YOGIC
BREATHING

We all breathe, but do we experience breathing? On each breath comes prana, the subtle life force, carried to us by the air. The prana that comes into us when we breathe is the same energy that animates all physical matter. By making the breath slow, deep, and conscious, we make the best use of the pranic energy. The result is that tension is released, calmness returns to the mind, and new awareness and insights are revealed which, in turn, uplift the consciousness.

Simple Yogic Breathing

All yogic breathing is done through the nose, unless otherwise specified.

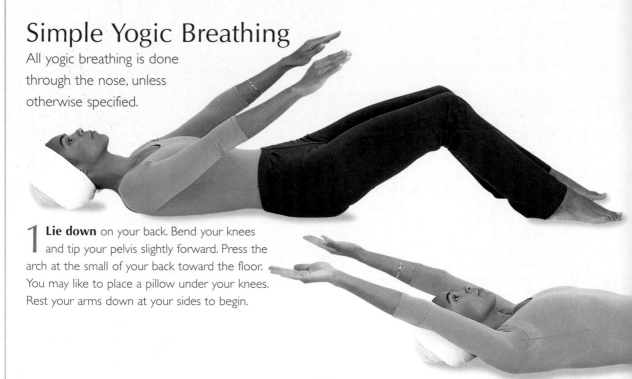

1 **Lie down** on your back. Bend your knees and tip your pelvis slightly forward. Press the arch at the small of your back toward the floor. You may like to place a pillow under your knees. Rest your arms down at your sides to begin.

Yogic Breathing Effects

• Increases the ability to use lung capacity through proper breathing.
• Develops the habit of breathing consciously, becoming aware of prana.
• Promotes the awareness of the inner connection with the universal consciousness.

2 **Inhalation** The inhalation has three parts that flow smoothly from one into the next. First, the diaphragm moves downward into the abdomen, drawing air into the lowest part of the lungs. Second, the rib cage expands and air is pulled into the middle part of the lungs. Lastly, the collarbones lift and air comes into the upper part of the chest. To help bring awareness to this process of deep breathing, use your arms as "monitors" for the inhalation process. As you begin to fill up the lower part of the lungs, raise the arms slowly from your sides. When you reach the mid-lungs, raise your arms to mirror that position. Continue raising your arms, smoothly mirroring the position of the breath in the lungs until they are full and the arms rest fully extended overhead.

Long Deep Breathing

Practice the simple yogic breathing sitting on the floor with a straight spine and the legs crossed. Your hands can be in Gian Mudra, Wisdom Pose, with the thumbs and index fingers forming a circle and the other fingers open. Straighten the arms. Relax the shoulders. Feel the natural flow of the breath.

By taking a deep yogic breath, you can expand the lungs to about 8 times their normal size. If you establish a habit of breathing deeply and slowly, you develop endurance and patience. If you slow the breath below 8 times per minute, the pituitary (located at the third-eye point or intuitive center) starts secreting fully. If the breath slows below 4 times per minute, the pineal gland (at the center of the skull) begins to function, and deep meditation is automatic.

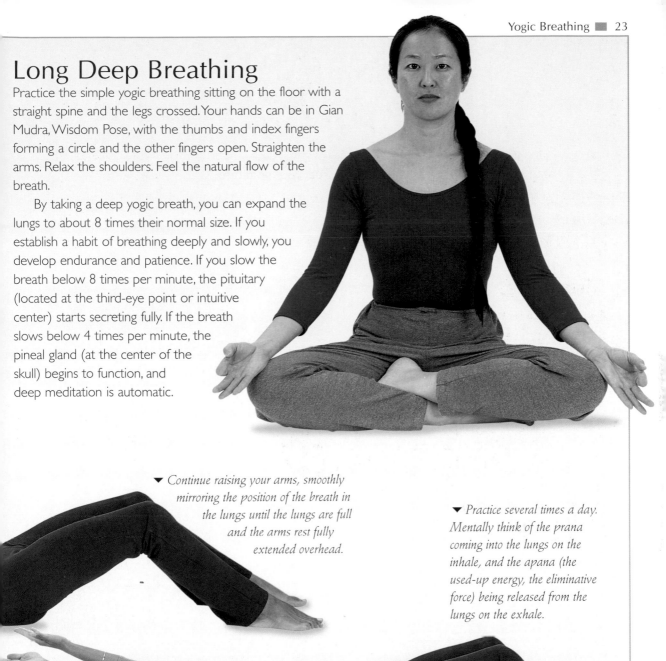

▼ *Continue raising your arms, smoothly mirroring the position of the breath in the lungs until the lungs are full and the arms rest fully extended overhead.*

▼ *Practice several times a day. Mentally think of the prana coming into the lungs on the inhale, and the apana (the used-up energy, the eliminative force) being released from the lungs on the exhale.*

3 **Exhalation** The process of exhalation in yogic breathing is the opposite of the inhalation. With arms overhead, begin to slowly exhale from the top part of the lungs first, moving your arms with the exhalation. The mid-lungs are emptied next, and the diaphragm moves upward as the last bit of air is emptied from the lungs and the arms come to rest at the sides once more.

PRANA-APANA
VISUALIZATION

Visualize the prana as light-energy entering you as you inhale. Feel it renewing your body, your mind, and your spirit. Feel your gratitude for this breath.

Now visualize the apana leaving as you exhale. See and feel the energy that has served you, but is no now longer needed. Bless it to leave you as you exhale. And welcome a new breath!

BREATH OF FIRE

This breath is used consistently throughout the Kundalini Yoga kriyas. The focal point of Breath of Fire is at the navel point. The breath is fairly rapid (2 to 3 breaths per second). It is continuous and powerful with no pause between the inhalation and exhalation. Breathe through the nose, unless directed otherwise. Here's how it works: As you exhale, the air is pushed out by pulling the navel point and abdomen toward the spine. As you inhale, release the inward pull of the navel to allow the breath to automatically return to the lungs. It may be helpful at first to put the hand on the abdomen to feel the inward pull on the exhalation, and the subsequent relaxation of the abdomen on the inhalation.

Although this is a very balanced breath with no emphasis on either the exhale or inhale, it may be helpful to focus primarily on the exhalation, which is synchronized with the pulling in of the navel. Listen to the sound of the breath, which will create the sound of a steam engine!

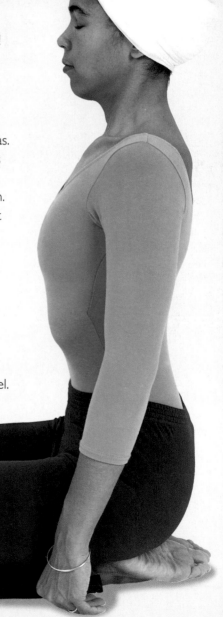

▶ *Pull the navel in towards the spine as you exhale.*

Breath of Fire is not hyperventilation. Hyperventilation could occur if one were using the upper chest to breathe rapidly. In Breath of Fire, the upper chest is held in suspension. Hyperventilation could also be caused by reversing Breath of Fire: exhaling with the navel pushed out, and inhaling with the navel pushed in. Look in a mirror if you are not certain of the movement, or place your hand on your abdomen, and go slowly.

Physical effects such as slight dizziness, slight headache, tickle, or tingle are normal, although not experienced by all. Since Breath of Fire is a purifying breath, toxins can be released into the bloodstream, especially in the beginning stages, causing symptoms such as the above. These effects will disappear after a time of consistent practice of Breath of Fire, and are not harmful.

Benefits of Breath of Fire

• Cleanses the blood, the mucous linings of the lungs, and all the cells.
• Expands the lung capacity.
• Strengthens all 72,000 nerves in the body.
• Warms up the body, and activates the brain. Studies show that Breath of Fire increases oxygen delivery to the brain, rejuvenating the brain's neurons.
• Adding Breath of Fire to an exercise shortens the time it takes to reach the desired effect.

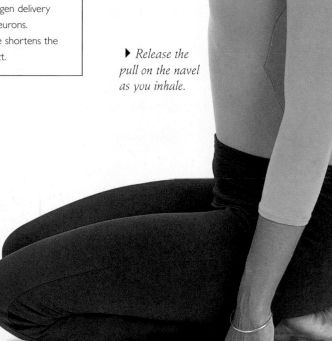

▶ *Release the pull on the navel as you inhale.*

SITALI BREATH

Sitali pranayam means "cooling breath." It soothes and cools the spine in the area of the fourth, fifth, and sixth vertebrae. This in turn regulates the sexual and digestive energy. This breath is often used for lowering fever and cooling off anger. This simple exercise rejuvenates and detoxifies when practiced regularly. Fifty-two breaths a day are recommended to extend your life span. Often the tongue tastes bitter at first. This is a sign of detoxification. As you continue the practice, the taste of the tongue will ultimately become sweet.

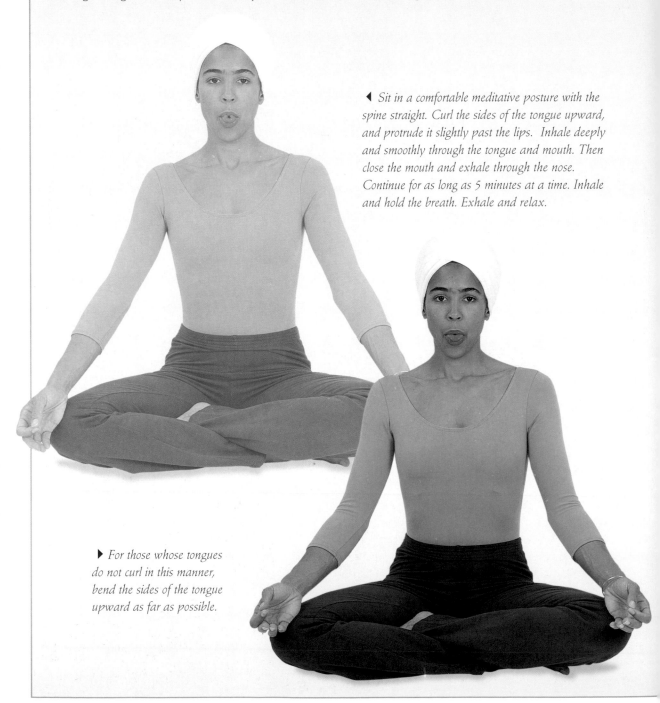

◀ *Sit in a comfortable meditative posture with the spine straight. Curl the sides of the tongue upward, and protrude it slightly past the lips. Inhale deeply and smoothly through the tongue and mouth. Then close the mouth and exhale through the nose. Continue for as long as 5 minutes at a time. Inhale and hold the breath. Exhale and relax.*

▶ *For those whose tongues do not curl in this manner, bend the sides of the tongue upward as far as possible.*

The right and left nostrils serve as regulators for your body temperature and your energy. The left nostril draws in the cooling, soothing, mind-expanding energy of the moon. The right nostril draws on the sun's energy for vitality, activity, and mental alertness. At any given moment one nostril is more open than the other. Your pituitary gland, which is considered by yogis to be the master gland, serves as the "thermostat" to control this. The switch between nostrils occurs naturally every 21/2 hours.

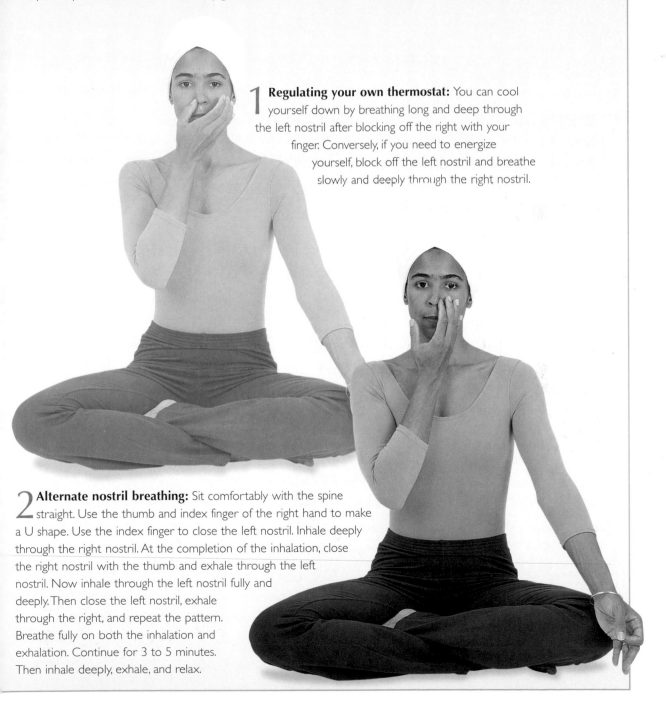

1 Regulating your own thermostat: You can cool yourself down by breathing long and deep through the left nostril after blocking off the right with your finger. Conversely, if you need to energize yourself, block off the left nostril and breathe slowly and deeply through the right nostril.

2 Alternate nostril breathing: Sit comfortably with the spine straight. Use the thumb and index finger of the right hand to make a U shape. Use the index finger to close the left nostril. Inhale deeply through the right nostril. At the completion of the inhalation, close the right nostril with the thumb and exhale through the left nostril. Now inhale through the left nostril fully and deeply. Then close the left nostril, exhale through the right, and repeat the pattern. Breathe fully on both the inhalation and exhalation. Continue for 3 to 5 minutes. Then inhale deeply, exhale, and relax.

ASANAS
SITTING POSES

Correct posture—keeping your spine straight—is an important factor in practicing sitting poses. Make sure the lower spine is straight, and the abdominal muscles are pulled in gently. The ribcage is slightly lifted, and the upper vertebrae are stacked on top of the lower vertebrae. Shoulders relax down and are gently pressed back in a natural way. The cervical vertebrae of the neck are straightened, and the neck stretches gently upward. The chin is parallel with the floor, and slightly tucked in. The head is in line with the spine. Feel as though there is an imaginary string that is strung through the lower, middle, and upper spine, the neck, and the top of the head. Imagine that this string is being gently tugged upward, straightening your posture in a gentle and natural way.

EASY POSES (SUKASANA)

Sit with the legs crossed. One foot is tucked inside, and the other is placed against the outside of the opposite leg. The knees are relaxed down toward the floor as far as possible. Straighten the lower spine.

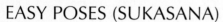

◀ The most common sitting pose in Kundalini Yoga and meditation is Easy Pose. This pose provides a firm and stable base for the body. It requires less flexibility and is easier on the knees than the Lotus Pose. There may be a tendency to slump in Easy Pose, so remain conscious of keeping the lower spine tipped slightly forward so that the upper spine can remain straight.

HALF LOTUS

Sit as above, then lift one foot and place it on the opposite thigh, as high as is comfortable. The foot will turn slightly so that the sole is facing upward. Straighten the lower spine.

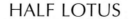

Lotus Pose (Padmasana)

Starting in Easy Pose, take hold of one foot with both hands and place it on your opposite thigh, as high as is comfortable. The foot will turn slightly so that the sole is facing upward. Next, take hold of the other foot and bring it up onto the opposite thigh. Keep the body erect with the head, neck, and chest in a straight line.

◀ *It is recommended that beginners start with Easy Pose and progress to Half-Lotus Pose before attempting Lotus. This classic sitting pose enhances concentration by automatically straightening the spine and providing a secure base. Once you are "locked into" Lotus, you can meditate deeply and the posture maintains itself.*

Rock Pose (Vajrasana)

Start by kneeling on both knees with the top of the feet on the ground. Sit back on the heels. The heels will press the two nerves that run into the lower center of each buttock, stimulating and activating them. Keep the spine pulled up straight.

▶ *This asana is well-known for its beneficial effects on the digestive system. It gained its name from the idea that one who masters this posture can sit in it and "digest rocks." It also makes you solid as a rock.*

Sitting in a Chair

If none of these poses are comfortable, it is possible to meditate in a chair. There are two important components for meditation in a chair: one, your back should stay as straight as possible; and two, to assure that the lower spine and hips are in balance, the feet need to be flat on the floor. If necessary, a firm pillow can be placed behind you to keep the back straight, or under the feet to keep them flat. There is a tendency to relax or slump in a chair. Be mindful of straightening the lower spine, feeling the vertebrae lined up properly, and keeping the neck straight with the chin slightly tucked. The hands can be in a meditative mudra. If you cannot sit on the floor, it is also possible to do some of the yoga and breathing exercises while sitting in a chair.

MUDRAS
HAND POSITIONS

Thousands of years ago, yogis mapped out the hand areas and their associated reflexes. Each area of the hand reflexes to a certain area of the body or brain. Each area also represents different emotions or behaviors. Mudras are hand positions that apply pressure on the different areas of the hands and fingers. Each mudra is a technique for giving clear messages to the mind/body energy system.

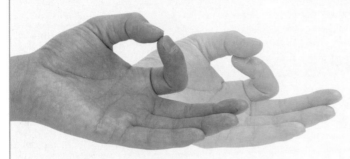

Gian Mudra

To form passive Gian Mudra, put the tip of the thumb together with the tip of the index finger. This stimulates knowledge and wisdom within you. It also increases receptivity and calmness.

To form active Gian Mudra, curl the index finger under the thumb so that the fingernail is against the joint of the thumb. This generates all of the same qualities as passive Gian Mudra, but with a more active, or projective energy.

▲ Gian Mudra increases wisdom and knowledge. It uses the index finger, which is represented by the planet Jupiter–the planet of expansion. This mudra is used with most meditative postures.

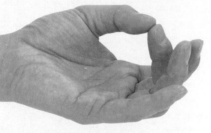

Shuni Mudra

Place the tip of the middle finger on the tip of the thumb. This gives patience, discernment, and the ability to commit

◀ Shuni Mudra increases patience and self-discipline. It uses the middle finger, which is represented by the planet Saturn–planet of responsibility, sometimes called the Task Master.

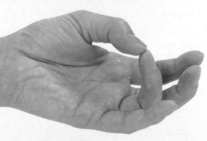

Surya Mudra

Place the tip of the ring finger on the tip of the thumb. Practicing this mudra gives revitalizing energy, nervous strength, and strong creativity.

◀ Practice Surya Mudra for energy. This pose uses the ring finger and is represented by the sun or Uranus. The sun gives energy; Uranus is the planet of intuition.

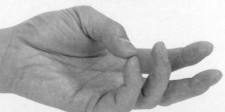

Buddhi Mudra

Place the tip of the little finger on the tip of the thumb. Practicing this mudra increases the capacity to communicate clearly and intuitively.

◀ Buddhi Mudra strengthens communication. It uses the little finger and is represented by the planet Mercury–the planet of mental power and communication.

Prayer Mudra

The positive side of the body (the right side, male), and the negative side (left, female) are neutralized by bringing the palms of the hands together and flat. Usually they are brought to the center of the chest at the heart level and the knuckles of the thumbs are pressed into the slight indentation at the sternum.

◀ Prayer Mudra can be used for invocation and devotion. It is always used when initially centering oneself in preparation for yoga (see "Before Beginning, Tune In" on page 44).

Venus Lock

Place the palms facing each other. For a woman, interlace the fingers with the right little finger on the bottom. Place the right thumb into the webbing between the thumb and index finger of the left hand. The tip of the left thumb presses the fleshy mound at the base of the right thumb. Positions are reversed for men.

▶ This mudra is used frequently in exercises. It derives its name from the fleshy mound at the base of the thumb, which is called the Venus mound. Pressure is applied to this mound by the thumb of the opposite hand. Venus is associated with love and sexuality. This mudra channels sexual energy and promotes glandular balance.

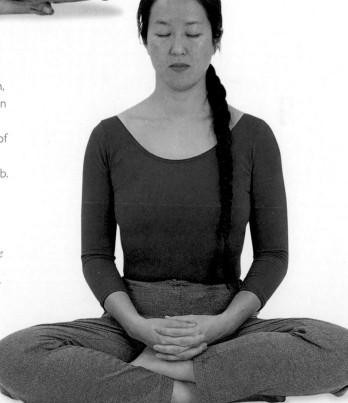

Bear Grip

Place the left palm facing out from the chest with the thumb down. Place the palm of the right hand facing the chest with the thumb up. Bring the fingers together. Curl the fingers of both hands so that the hands form a fist.

▶ *This mudra is used to stimulate the heart and intensify concentration. It is often practiced with a held inhalation or exhalation, while pulling the lock with as much strength as possible.*

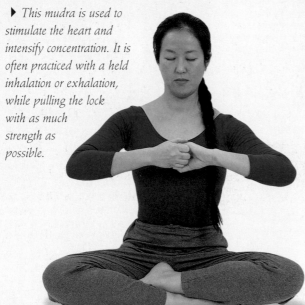

Hands In Lap Mudras

Fingers interlaced: Interlace the fingers and place them in your lap with the palms facing upward. Thumbs may be relaxed, or the tips may touch each other.

Palms resting: For a man, rest the left hand in the lap with the right hand on top of it. Both palms face upward. Put the thumb tips together. The hand positions are reversed for women.

▶ *This mudra is a relaxed and receptive hand position for meditation.*

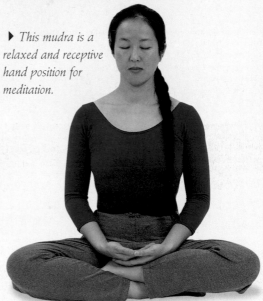

Using a Mala

A mala is a closed string design with a calculated number of beads (usually 108, 54, or 27). As your first finger and thumb touch each bead, repeat the mantra either mentally or orally. Rotate the mala through the fingers, and when you reach the "guru bead," which is larger, twist the mala around and begin again, returning in the same direction you started from. This is one round.

In addition to assisting in the repetition of mantra, the mala stimulates the nervous system and brain through the reflex points activated by the continual pressing of the fingertips on the beads. (See "Resources" for where to obtain a mala.)

The most commonly used mantra in Kundalini Yoga is *Sat Nam* (rhymes with "but mom"). It is called the bij (seed) mantra. The literal meaning of *Sat Nam* is "Truth is my Identity" or "Truth-Identity." It is comprised of the syllables *sa ta na ma*, which are among the most elemental sounds of creation. By saying *Sat Nam* as a greeting, you are reinforcing the highest consciousness in yourself and everyone you meet. By hearing *Sat Nam* silently on the breath, you remind yourself that you are truth manifested. And by chanting *Sat Nam*, you experience the truth of what you are chanting. (See chapter 7, "Meditation," for how to practice this and other mantras.)

MANTRA
THE YOGA
OF SOUND

The word mantra translates as "mind projection." It is a technique for regulating the mind. There are many mantras, each one having its own quality, rhythm, and effect. In Kundalini Yoga, an individualized, "secret" mantra is not given. All mantras can be learned and used by anyone.

Our world is made up of energy. Energy vibrates. Some energy, like an inanimate object, vibrates slower, or at a lower frequency. Some energy, like a thought, vibrates at a rate we cannot see. Experiencing energy that vibrates at a higher frequency brings us closer to merging with the highest vibration of all, which is sometimes called God.

Every thought or feeling we have is on a vibratory frequency. By using mantras we direct the mind into a high vibratory frequency. Mantra yoga is a technique of yoking the individual with the whole. This is accomplished by merging the sound vibration of the individual consciousness with that of the universal consciousness through the rhythmic power of the mantra.

How It Works

The total effect of mantra depends on the reflex points on the tongue and in the mouth. On the roof of the mouth there are 84 meridian, or pressure, points. Every time you speak, you stimulate them with the tongue. When you press the right "codes," it sends messages to the brain to unlock the higher centers. Mantras contain the ancient technology to send these codes to the brain.

The sound of the mantra can be directed to resonate from several areas of the body, the most common being the third-eye point. By directing your eyes, or your attention, to that area and chanting the sound, you vibrate the mantra at the third-eye point. Other centers that are often used are the navel center, the heart center, and the crown center at the top of the head.

When we chant, which is more like vibrating a sound than singing, we are consciously directing the mind. We are choosing to invoke the positive power contained within those sounds.

Positive affirmations spoken in one's own language are also effective tools of transformation. They are a form of mantra that positively affect the mind.

Ultimately the practice of mantra is perfected so that all mantra is *japa*. *Japa* means "to resound the mantra." In *japa*, the mantra is projected to the cosmos and then reflected back to you. When *japa* is mastered, you can hear the mantra without feeling that you produced it.

This *japa* leads to *tapa*, the inner psychic heat of prana. *Tapa* cleans and strengthens the nerves. The practice of *japa* is often done with the aid of a string of beads know as a *mala*.

BANDHAS
BODY LOCKS

Bandhas, or body locks, are certain combinations of muscle contractions. Each lock functions to change blood circulation, nerve pressure, and the flow of cerebral spinal fluid. They also direct the flow of prana (life force) into the main energy channels that relate to raising the kundalini energy. They help concentrate the body's energy for use in raising consciousness and self-healing. There are three important locks in Kundalini Yoga: Neck Lock, Diaphragm Lock, and Root Lock.

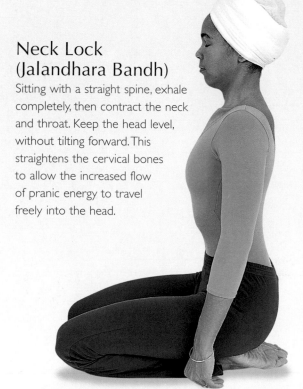

Neck Lock (Jalandhara Bandh)

Sitting with a straight spine, exhale completely, then contract the neck and throat. Keep the head level, without tilting forward. This straightens the cervical bones to allow the increased flow of pranic energy to travel freely into the head.

▲ *The Neck Lock helps the thyroid and parathyroid glands to secrete optimally and helps activate the higher functions of the pituitary. In the Kundalini Yoga kriyas, powerful energy is generated; as it moves through the channels, it can meet with some blocks. When this blocking happens, there can sometimes be a quick shift in blood pressure, causing dizziness. This can be avoided by applying the Neck Lock.*

Diaphragm Lock (Uddiyana Bandh)

Sit with a straight spine and exhale all breath. Pull the upper abdominal muscles back toward the spine and lift the diaphragm up high into the thorax. Diaphragm Lock is normally applied on the exhalation. Applying it forcefully on the inhalation can over-pressurize the eyes and heart.

▲ *The Diaphragm Lock gives a gentle massage to the heart muscles. It allows the pranic force to move through the central nerve channel of the spine and up into the neck region. It stimulates the proper functioning of the hypothalamus, pituitary, and adrenal glands. Regular use of the Diaphragm Lock brings youthfulness and a sense of compassion. Use of this lock during chanting enhances the effects.*

Root Lock
(Mul Bandh)

First exhale, then contract the anal muscle and draw it in and up. Add to that a contraction of the sexual organ. Lastly, pull in the navel by drawing back the lower abdomen toward the spine. The rectum and sex organs will be drawn up toward the navel point. The Root Lock is usually applied at the end of a deep exhalation, and released on the subsequent inhalation. As you inhale, focus on energy moving up the spine; end your inhalation by concentrating either on the third-eye point or the crown center. Infrequently, the instructions for certain poses will specify to apply the Root Lock on the held inhalation, and release on the following exhalation.

▲ *The Root Lock, or Mul Bandh, is frequently applied in Kundalini Yoga. Mul is the "root, base or source." The action of the Root Lock unites the two major energy flows of the body: prana and apana. Prana is the inflowing life source, the generative energy of the upper body and heart center. Apana is the downward flow of eliminative energy. The Root Lock pulls the apana up and the prana down to mix at the navel center. This combination generates the "heat" that can release the kundalini energy.*

To strengthen the Root Lock muscles and help avoid incontinence later in life, add this daily practice: when you eliminate, stop the flow of urine with your internal muscles, and then relax the flow. Practice a few times a day.

The Great Lock
(Maha Bandh)

This is the application of all three body locks at one time, starting with the Root Lock, adding the Diaphragm Lock, and then the Neck Lock. Usually this lock is applied at the end of a deep exhale, and released on the following inhale.

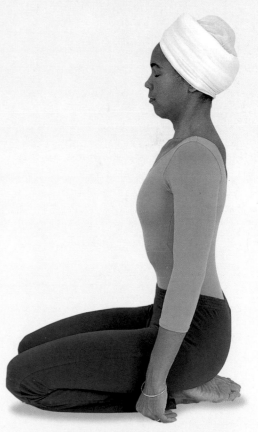

▲ *The Maha Bandh rejuvenates the nerves and glands. The practice and perfection of this lock is said to relieve preoccupation with sex. It helps circulate blood into the reproductive glands, and is an overall tonic to the male and female sexual organs.*

CHAKRAS
ENERGY CENTERS

Kundalini Yoga is a tool we use to activate and transform the body's energy centers, called chakras. It is, therefore, essential to understand the chakras and become aware of the role they play in our lives.

The body is made up of fields of energy that most of us cannot see with our eyes. Those who can, say that these fields of energy are like fluid whirlpools of light that are constantly moving and changing in complex patterns. The yogic name for these centers is chakras, literally "circles" in Sanskrit.

There are seven major chakras that interact with the body, and one that encompasses them all, totaling eight. Even though they are mostly unseen, our chakras interact with and influence our thoughts, moods, and health. Energy flows through the entire body from the chakras. Six chakras are located in the body, the seventh is at the top of the skull, and the eighth is the aura, or magnetic field, that surrounds the entire body. All the main chakras are connected by a channel of energy called the shushmana that travels up the center of the spine and around the brain.

Each chakra has an important function to perform for us, and we need all of them. The first, second, and third chakras are sometimes referred to as the "lower triangle" or the lower chakras, but they are just as important as the "upper triangle" or higher centers. The first three chakras deal mainly with the physical needs of the body and basic needs of life. The last five work within the spiritual realms and are rooted in universal consciousness.

Kundalini Yoga and the Chakras

We practice Kundalini Yoga in order to balance and coordinate the functions of the lower chakras and to experience the realms of the higher chakras. After the kundalini energy rises and becomes accustomed to flowing freely through all the chakras, there is a definite change of consciousness, a noticeable transformation in the character of an individual. The person looks at life differently, feels different and therefore acts differently. The real "proof" that someone's kundalini has risen lies in the upgrading of that person's attitude toward life, his relationships with other people and with himself.

–Shakti Parwha Kaur Khalsa
Kundalini Yoga: The Flow of Eternal Power

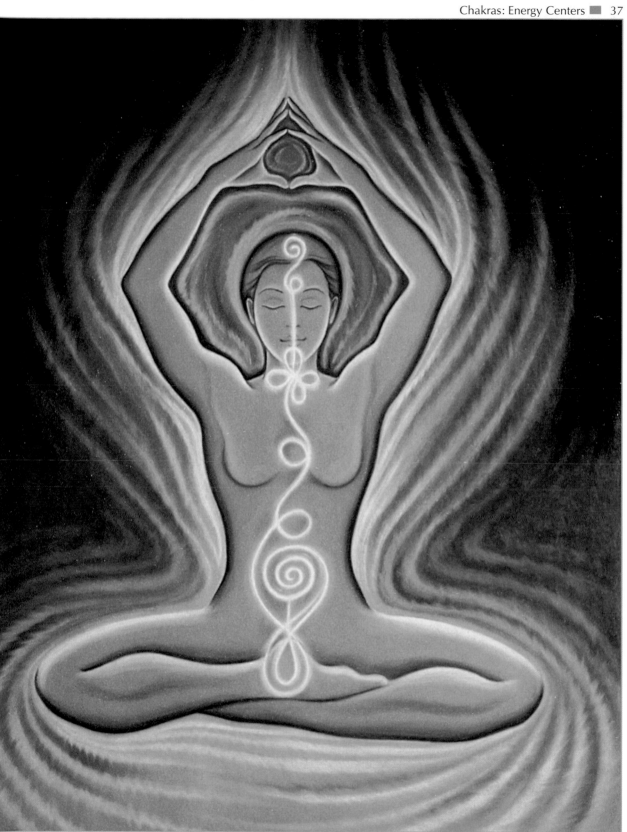

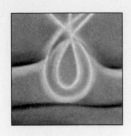

FIRST CHAKRA:

Located at the rectum and base of the spine at the conjunction of 72,000 nerve endings.

Function: This chakra works to eliminate solid waste. Its concerns are of basic survival and security.

In an imbalance of the first chakra, fear, perversion, and insecurity dominate. When balanced, this chakra brings strength and confidence.

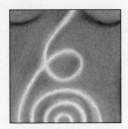

SECOND CHAKRA:

Located at the third and fourth vertebra and sex organs.

Function: The second chakra controls sex and reproduction, as well as mental creativity.

Imbalances in the second chakra bring obsession with sex or unhealthy indulgence of fantasy. When balanced, one is creative, imaginative, energized, and has a balanced sexual life.

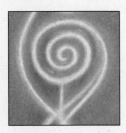

THIRD CHAKRA:

Located at the navel point where all nerve endings meet.

Function: The third chakra controls the fire of digestion. Its primary concerns are those of identity, domain, and judgment.

When in a state of imbalance, the third chakra can manifest as excessive greed or an overwhelming drive for personal power. A weak navel chakra can bring susceptibility to illness. A strong navel can give good physical health. When in balance, it gives the initiative and courage to persevere and accomplish great deeds.

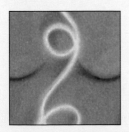

FOURTH CHAKRA:

Located at the "heart center" which is in the center of the chest, not at the physical heart and is associated with the thymus gland.

Function: The heart center is the balance point between the lower chakras and the higher chakras. When the heart chakra becomes active, true love can be experienced. It is the center for kindness, compassion, and selfless acts of giving. In an imbalance, acting from the emotions can be confused with acting from the heart center. Feelings and emotions are sensory, and stem from the second chakra, whereas the fourth chakra consciously channels those emotions into devotion, and passion into compassion.

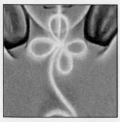

FIFTH CHAKRA:

The fifth chakra is located at the throat and is associated with the thyroid gland.

Function: The fifth chakra monitors the power and impact of speech. Words that penetrate and project come from a strong fifth chakra.

An imbalance can result in blunt or highly opinionated communication. In balance, the fifth chakra is concerned with speaking truth in the highest sense.

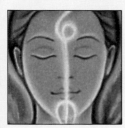

SIXTH CHAKRA:

Located at the center of the forehead, slightly above the eyebrows, and associated with the pituitary gland. It is sometimes referred to as the "third eye" or "third-eye point."

Function: This is where we can "see the unseen, and know the unknown." It is the center of our sense of intuition, and our direct connection to the infinite source of wisdom.

Frequent activation of the sixth chakra through meditation increases pituitary gland secretion, and allows us to become more intuitive. Being intuitive is not the same as being psychic. Psychic powers use energy from and function through the third chakra, and can therefore be subjective.

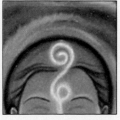

SEVENTH CHAKRA:

Located at the top of the skull and associated with the pineal gland. The seventh chakra is also referred to as the "Thousand-Petaled Lotus," the "Tenth Gate," and the "Crown Chakra."

Function: This is the highest center located within the body. When the kundalini energy is raised to the seventh chakra, one experiences a state of bliss, a union with the cosmos.

It is said that when an enlightened soul leaves the body, it leaves through the seventh chakra.

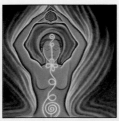

EIGHTH CHAKRA:

The energy field that surrounds the entire body. It is also called the aura.

Function: The aura is the protective shield that encloses the other chakras. It changes in color, brightness, and size depending on your general physical health and your thoughts and feelings.

The aura normally extends several feet in every direction, and can grow brighter and larger with consistent healthy body/mind/spirit practices, such as Kundalini Yoga and meditation.

KRIYAS

The word kriya literally means "action." It is an action which "must sprout the seed," in the words of Yogi Bhajan. In Kundalini Yoga, it is an exercise or group of exercises that work toward a specific outcome. Every exercise is not a kriya. Practicing a kriya initiates a sequence of physical and mental changes that affect the body, mind, and spirit simultaneously. Each kriya has a different effect, but all work on all levels of your being.

Some kriyas, such as Sat Kriya, are a single exercise/meditation, while others are complete exercise sets. Included here are two powerful single-exercise kriyas.

Sat Kriya

Stretch the arms up with the elbows hugging the sides of the head. Interlock all the fingers except the index fingers of each hand, which are pointing straight up. Begin to say the sound *sat* (rhymes with "but") as you pull the navel up and in toward the spine. The sound should be very powerful but not necessarily loud. As you say *nam* (rhymes with "mom"), relax the belly area. *Nam* is short, the syllable is not extended. It may be barely audible. Chant emphatically in a constant rhythm about 8 times per 10 seconds. Then, inhale and squeeze the muscles tightly from the buttocks all the way up the back, past the shoulders. Mentally allow the energy to flow through the head and out the top of the skull. Hold for 5 to 10 seconds. Exhale and relax.

◀ *Sat Kriya is fundamental to Kundalini Yoga, and it is good to practice it every day for at least 3 minutes. It strengthens the entire sexual system and eliminative system. General physical health is improved since all the internal organs receive a gentle rhythmic massage from this exercise.*

Sat Kriya works directly on stimulating and channeling the kundalini energy, so to keep the energy focused and pure, always chant Sat Nam while performing it. Beginners should practice Sat Kriya for 1 minute, working up slowly to 3 minutes. After a time of steady practice, the length of Sat Kriya can be extended, but remember to approach this powerful kriya with respect. Those who have been practicing Kundalini Yoga for many years and have been drug- and chemical-free for at least a few years can eventually begin to do Sat Kriya with both hands pressed flat against each other. This releases more energy, but must be used cautiously.

Ideally you should relax for at least the same amount of time as you practice Sat Kriya; it is recommended that you relax for up to twice that amount of time. Relax either in Gurpranam Pose or on the back in Corpse Pose.

Gurpranam Pose

While sitting on the heels, bring the forehead to the floor and stretch the arms forward with the palms together. The outside edge of the hands will rest on the floor.

▼ *This brings not only relaxation, but also an active sense of "knowing." It calls on the Gur, "Infinite Wisdom." It is said that in ancient times the master would instruct the disciple to stay in Gurpranam Pose for long periods of time, sometimes for days. At the end of that time, the disciple would understand the answer to the question he had come to ask the master.*

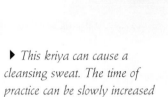

▶ *This kriya can cause a cleansing sweat. The time of practice can be slowly increased up to 7½ minutes on each side.*

▶ *The practice and perfection of this kriya is said to activate pituitary secretion, regulate excessive sexual energy, and increase general immunity to disease. The nerves are strengthened, and the magnetic field of the body is returned to balance. If you do not want to be shaky when you are older, practice this while you are younger.*

Varuyas Kriya

Stand up straight. Put the right foot slightly forward. Stretch the left leg far back, but keep your balance. Put the top of the toes of the left foot on the ground. Extend the arms forward, parallel to the ground. Put the palms together so that the fingers point away from you. The spine is extended slightly forward. Fix the eyes on the horizon or at the brow point (third-eye point). Take a deep breath, then begin a rhythmic chant of *Sat Nam*. Emphasize the sound sat as you pull the navel point in and apply a light Root Lock. Continue for 1 minute. Then inhale, exhale, and relax. Switch and place the left leg forward. Repeat the exercise for an equal period of time.

CHAPTER 3

WARMING UP TO YOGA

"Whether you call it serpent power, kundalini, the power of Soul Consciousness, or Divine Consciousness, the gift of this divine energy gives a person equilibrium. You must remember that whenever your mind is in a state of equilibrium, you will be radiant. Your spirit will rise like the tide rises. When the moon is near the Earth, there is a high tide. The same thing happens to the spirit in a person."
–*Yogi Bhajan*

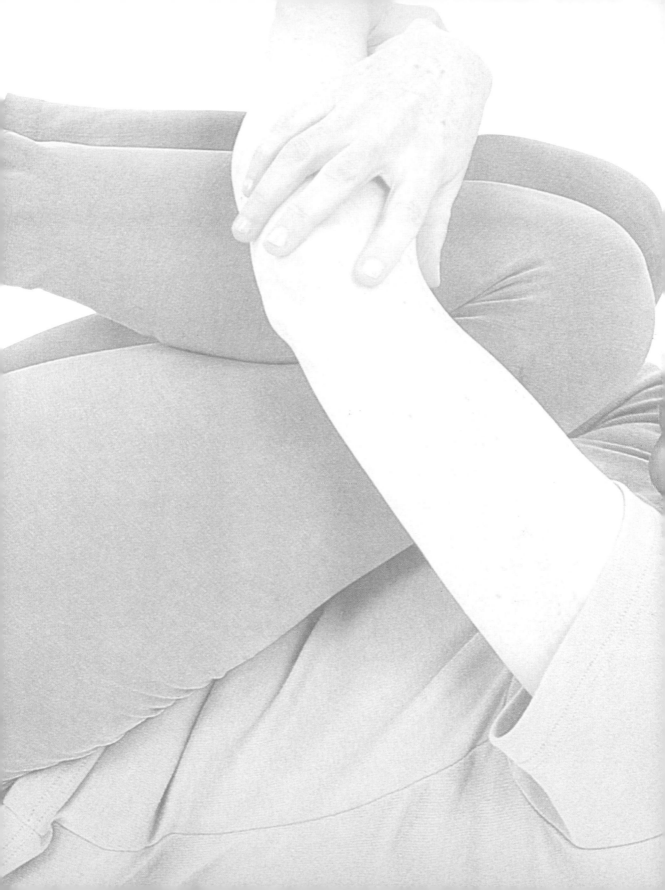

BEFORE BEGINNING
TUNE IN

In Kundalini Yoga a sound vibration (mantra) is used to connect with both the higher self and the lineage of this ancient science. According to yogic knowledge, when a sound's innate vibration corresponds to or in some way reproduces what it refers to, it is a sacred language. This is the underlying principle in languages such as Sanskrit and Gurmukhi. Chanting these ancient syllables is the fastest possible path to vibratory union between ourselves and the universal consciousness.

ONG NAMO GURU DEV NAMO

Ong is the infinite creative energy. It is a variation of the cosmic syllable *Om*, which denotes the Absolute, the Hidden Creator. In the functioning, creative state, it becomes *ong*. To chant *ong*, slightly pull in the navel and vibrate the *ng* at the root of the nose.

Namo (pronounced nah-moe) has the same root as the word *nameste*, which means "reverent greetings" or "I bow to you."

Together, *Ong Namo* means, "I call on the infinite creative consciousness."

Guru is the teacher or the embodiment of wisdom. *Gu* means darkness, and *ru* means light, so *Guru* means "that which takes one from darkness to light." The first syllable, *gu*, is short, while the second, *ru*, is long (pronounced together as g'roo). The *r* is rolled off the roof of the mouth.

Dev means transparent, or non-physical (pronounced like Dave). And repeat *namo* once again.

Together, *Guru Dev Namo* means, "I call on the divine teacher, or the universal wisdom."

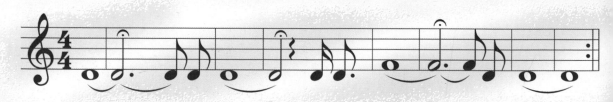

ong...   namo...   guru dev...   namo...

The Importance of Warming-up

As you look through this book you will find many yoga sets, or kriyas, that work on specific areas of the body and mind. Many of them require an already warmed-up and flexible body. It is recommended that you first do at least some of the exercises given on the next pages. Start with warming the base of the spine, and work your way upward, including stretching the sciatic nerve in the legs. It is recommended that you spend between 10 and 15 minutes with warm-ups before choosing a specific yoga set.

It is essential to create an internal awareness during yoga, not only to reap the greatest benefits, but also to prevent injury to the body. As best you can, apply your meditative mind to each moment spent in Kundalini Yoga. Feel the

difference between a "good" hurt and a "bad" hurt. A "good" hurt feels like a muscle offering resistance, then relaxing and unwinding. To encourage this process, link your breath with the mental focus of mantra (*Sat* on the inhale and *Nam* on the exhale is most commonly used) and visualize yourself relaxing more deeply. A "bad" hurt feels like a muscle overstretching before it is ready to. Of course, use common sense. As with any exercise program, caution and common sense must be used if you have medical problems.

It is recommended for beginners in Kundalini Yoga to start with the minimum times given, gradually increasing the time as the practice progresses.

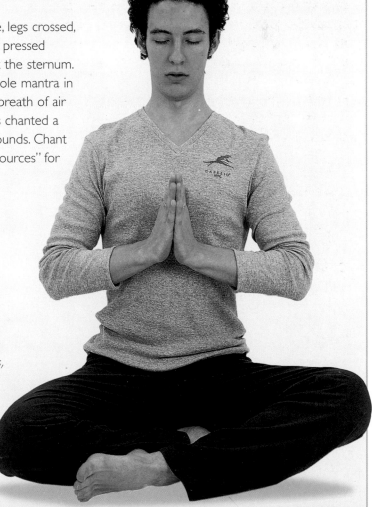

To chant this mantra, sit with a straight spine, legs crossed, and eyes closed. The palms of the hands are pressed together, and the joints of the thumbs are at the sternum. Take a deep breath and either chant the whole mantra in one breath, or chant *Ong Namo*, take a half breath of air and chant *Guru Dev Namo*. The sound *Dev* is chanted a minor third interval higher than the other sounds. Chant the entire mantra at least 3 times. (See "Resources" for companion CD with this mantra.)

▶ *This mantra–called the Adi (primal, original) Mantra–is chanted or vibrated at least 3 times at the onset of each Kundalini Yoga practice or class, in order to assure the purest inner guidance. It is the "golden link" to the long line of spiritual masters of Kundalini Yoga who have preceded us. Yogi Bhajan is the immediate connection to this chain of masters. The Adi Mantra opens the protective channel of energy for Kundalini Yoga.*

SERIES TO
ENERGIZE

These 3 exercises can be done before you get out of bed in the morning, or as the first exercises of your yoga routine.

STRETCH POSE

Stretch the legs forward, raise the arms over your head, and stretch like a cat. Arch the spine and flex all of your muscles both left and right. Then tip the pelvis forward, bring the feet together and raise them 6 inches from the ground, keeping the legs straight. Raise your head 6 inches and fix your eyes on the toes, which point away from you. Arms are held straight at the sides, palms facing the thighs but not touching. Hold this position for 1 minute with Breath of Fire. Relax for a few seconds.

▼ *Stretch Pose adjusts the navel point. Since the navel is the focal point for all 72,000 nerves in the body, Stretch Pose tunes up the whole nervous system as well as the digestive and reproductive systems.*

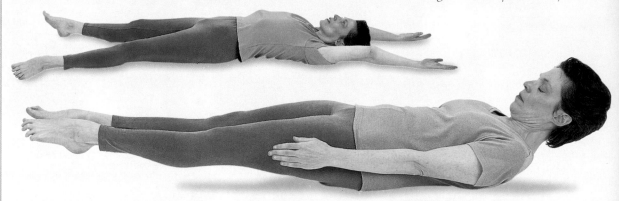

NOSE TO KNEES POSE

Bend the knees to the chest, wrap the arms around them, and press them tightly to the chest. Bring your head up so that the nose comes as close to the knees as possible. Do Breath of Fire for 30 seconds to 1 minute. Inhale and stretch. Then exhale and relax down for a few seconds.

▶ *This exercise stimulates the apana (eliminative life force), helping the body cleanse and eliminate toxins.*

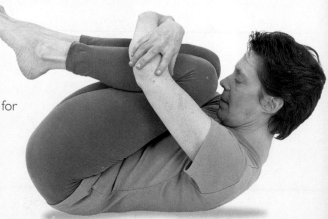

EGO ERADICATOR

Rock back and forth on the spine a few times with the knees pulled to the chest and the arms wrapped around the legs. Come to a squatting position either on or between the heels. Bring the arms out to the sides, and raise them until they form a V shape. Stretch the thumbs up toward the sky. The rest of the fingers are curled onto the pads directly below the fingers. Begin a powerful Breath of Fire.

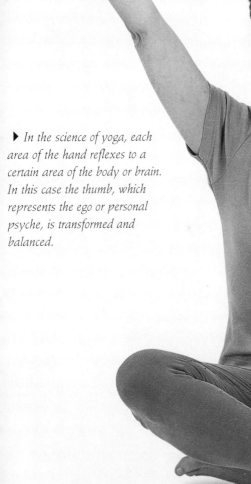

▶ *In the science of yoga, each area of the hand reflexes to a certain area of the body or brain. In this case the thumb, which represents the ego or personal psyche, is transformed and balanced.*

SPINAL
WARM-UPS

The following exercises prepare the body, and specifically the spine, for the kriyas given in this book. They need not all be done each time. They should warm the spine systematically from the base of the spine upward.

1 **Lower Spine Flex** Start by sitting on the floor with the legs crossed and tucked in. Straighten the spine by pressing the chest slightly forward and lifting the ribcage. Relax the shoulders and slightly tuck the chin. This is sitting in Easy Pose. Now take hold of the outside ankle with both hands. Inhale and flex the spine forward, chest out and shoulders back. Exhale and slump the body, keeping the chin level.

▶ *This exercise loosens the vertebrae of the lower spine and stimulates the energy there.*

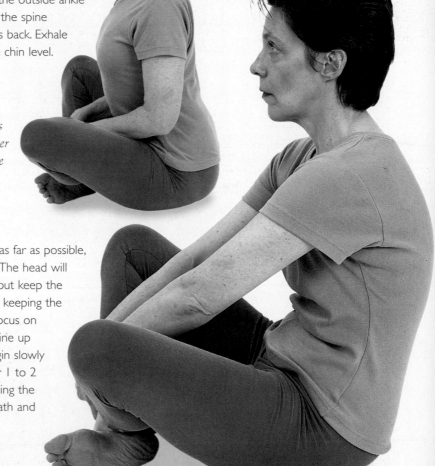

2 Exhale and slump the spine as far as possible, shoulders rounded forward. The head will come forward to some degree, but keep the focus on rounding the spine and keeping the chin level as much as possible. Focus on flexing the area from the mid-spine up through the shoulder blades. Begin slowly and pick up the pace. Repeat for 1 to 2 minutes. Then inhale deeply, holding the breath. Exhale and relax the breath and the pose.

Waist Rolls Still sitting in Easy Pose, place your hands on your knees. As you inhale, begin a deep roll of the waist and hips to the right, then to the back. Exhale as you roll around to the left and front. Continue for 1 minute. Then reverse the direction so you are inhaling as you roll to the left and the back; then exhaling as you come around to the right. Continue in this direction for 1 minute. Deepen the circles as you go.

◀ *The energy of the lower spine is moved upward in this exercise. Waist Rolls also strengthen the digestive system and the muscles of the waist and back.*

1 **Upper Spine Flex** Sitting in Easy Pose, grasp the knees with the hands. Inhale and pull your body forward. The chest will be lifted and the shoulders stretched back.

◀ *The vertebrae of the mid-spine are flexed, and digestion is stimulated. Energy is circulated in the mid- and upper back.*

2 Exhale and slump the spine as far as possible, shoulders rounded forward. Keep the elbows straight. Focus your awareness on the area from the mid-spine up through the shoulder blades. Again, feel each vertebra flexing as you move. Begin slowly and pick up the pace as you continue for 1 to 2 minutes. Inhale deeply and stretch. Then exhale and relax the breath.

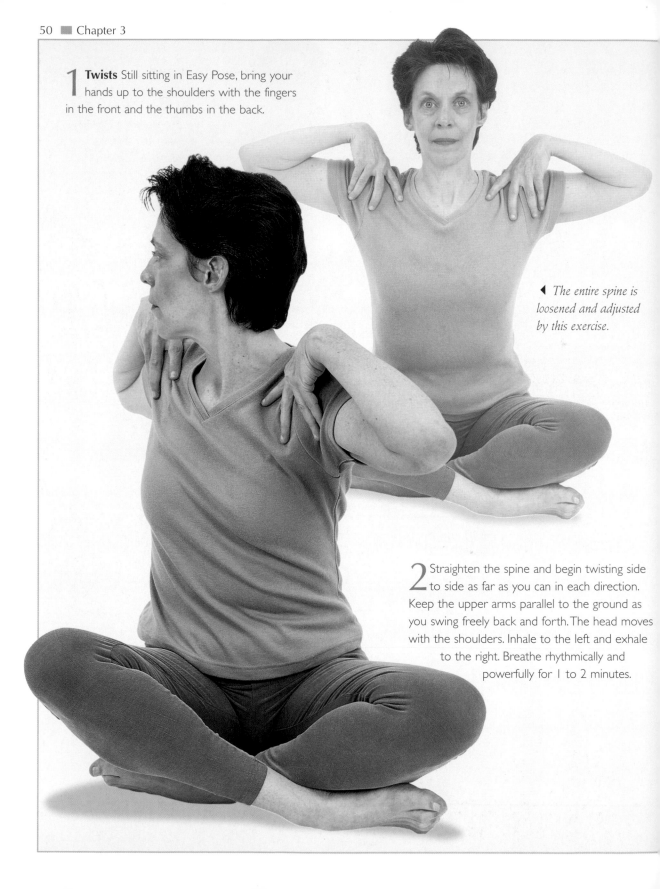

1 **Twists** Still sitting in Easy Pose, bring your hands up to the shoulders with the fingers in the front and the thumbs in the back.

◀ *The entire spine is loosened and adjusted by this exercise.*

2 Straighten the spine and begin twisting side to side as far as you can in each direction. Keep the upper arms parallel to the ground as you swing freely back and forth. The head moves with the shoulders. Inhale to the left and exhale to the right. Breathe rhythmically and powerfully for 1 to 2 minutes.

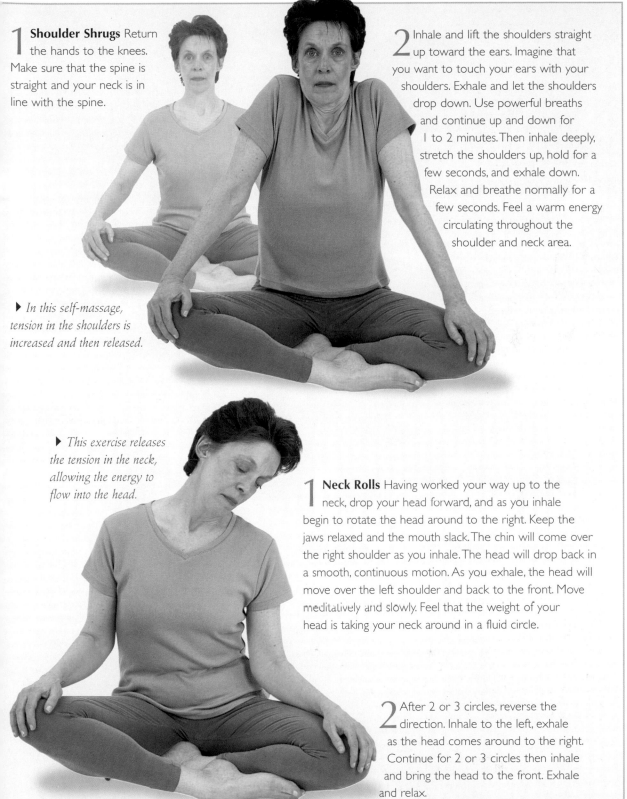

1 **Shoulder Shrugs** Return the hands to the knees. Make sure that the spine is straight and your neck is in line with the spine.

2 Inhale and lift the shoulders straight up toward the ears. Imagine that you want to touch your ears with your shoulders. Exhale and let the shoulders drop down. Use powerful breaths and continue up and down for 1 to 2 minutes. Then inhale deeply, stretch the shoulders up, hold for a few seconds, and exhale down. Relax and breathe normally for a few seconds. Feel a warm energy circulating throughout the shoulder and neck area.

▶ *In this self-massage, tension in the shoulders is increased and then released.*

▶ *This exercise releases the tension in the neck, allowing the energy to flow into the head.*

1 **Neck Rolls** Having worked your way up to the neck, drop your head forward, and as you inhale begin to rotate the head around to the right. Keep the jaws relaxed and the mouth slack. The chin will come over the right shoulder as you inhale. The head will drop back in a smooth, continuous motion. As you exhale, the head will move over the left shoulder and back to the front. Move meditatively and slowly. Feel that the weight of your head is taking your neck around in a fluid circle.

2 After 2 or 3 circles, reverse the direction. Inhale to the left, exhale as the head comes around to the right. Continue for 2 or 3 circles then inhale and bring the head to the front. Exhale and relax.

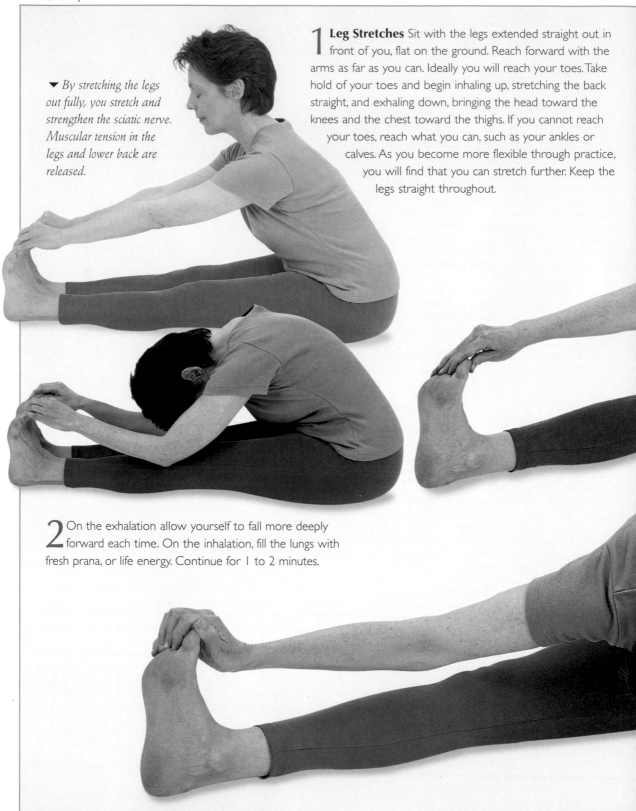

▼ *By stretching the legs out fully, you stretch and strengthen the sciatic nerve. Muscular tension in the legs and lower back are released.*

1 Leg Stretches Sit with the legs extended straight out in front of you, flat on the ground. Reach forward with the arms as far as you can. Ideally you will reach your toes. Take hold of your toes and begin inhaling up, stretching the back straight, and exhaling down, bringing the head toward the knees and the chest toward the thighs. If you cannot reach your toes, reach what you can, such as your ankles or calves. As you become more flexible through practice, you will find that you can stretch further. Keep the legs straight throughout.

2 On the exhalation allow yourself to fall more deeply forward each time. On the inhalation, fill the lungs with fresh prana, or life energy. Continue for 1 to 2 minutes.

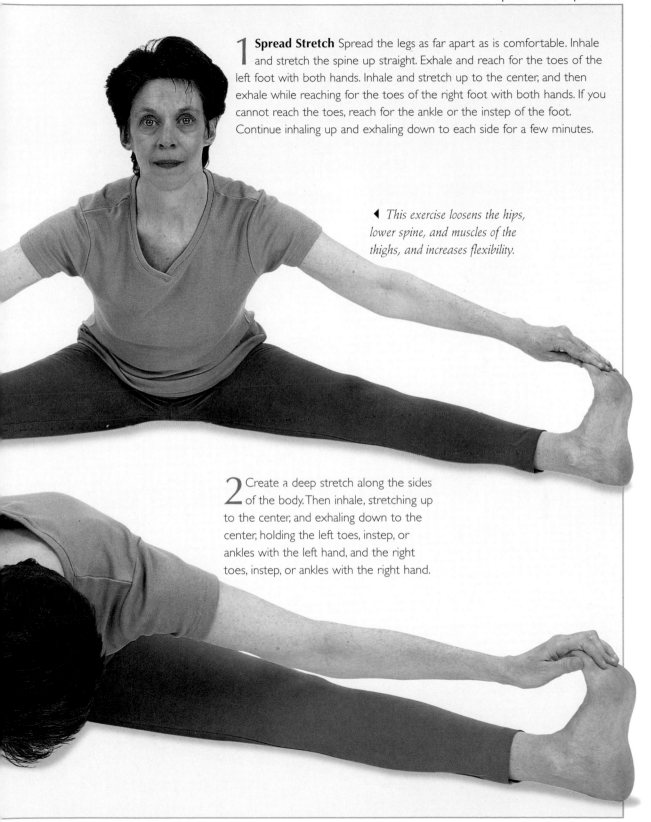

1 **Spread Stretch** Spread the legs as far apart as is comfortable. Inhale and stretch the spine up straight. Exhale and reach for the toes of the left foot with both hands. Inhale and stretch up to the center, and then exhale while reaching for the toes of the right foot with both hands. If you cannot reach the toes, reach for the ankle or the instep of the foot. Continue inhaling up and exhaling down to each side for a few minutes.

◀ *This exercise loosens the hips, lower spine, and muscles of the thighs, and increases flexibility.*

2 Create a deep stretch along the sides of the body. Then inhale, stretching up to the center, and exhaling down to the center, holding the left toes, instep, or ankles with the left hand, and the right toes, instep, or ankles with the right hand.

EVERYDAY
YOGA POSES

Here are some of the most commonly used Kundalini Yoga exercises. Choose from them to extend your warm-up routine, or practice them before any of the yoga sets found in this book. Practice them for 1 to 2 minutes each with deep breathing or Breath of Fire.

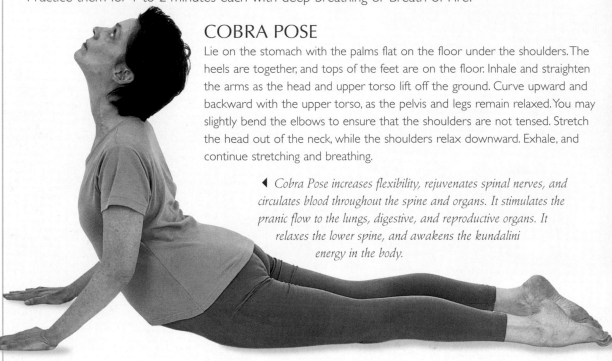

COBRA POSE

Lie on the stomach with the palms flat on the floor under the shoulders. The heels are together, and tops of the feet are on the floor. Inhale and straighten the arms as the head and upper torso lift off the ground. Curve upward and backward with the upper torso, as the pelvis and legs remain relaxed. You may slightly bend the elbows to ensure that the shoulders are not tensed. Stretch the head out of the neck, while the shoulders relax downward. Exhale, and continue stretching and breathing.

◄ *Cobra Pose increases flexibility, rejuvenates spinal nerves, and circulates blood throughout the spine and organs. It stimulates the pranic flow to the lungs, digestive, and reproductive organs. It relaxes the lower spine, and awakens the kundalini energy in the body.*

VARIATION

Cobra Curl-ups Lie on the stomach. Place the hands on the floor, a little closer to the chest than in the previous Cobra Pose, and stretch up into Cobra while inhaling. Exhale while you lift the buttocks, and press them back into the heels. As you tuck your body back, bring the forehead to the ground and keep the hands where they were (this is Baby Pose), giving the upper body and spine a good stretch. Then continue inhaling into Cobra Pose and exhaling into Baby Pose. Continue for 1 to 2 minutes.

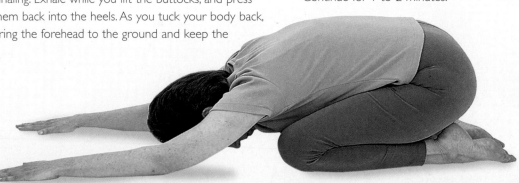

CAMEL POSE

Kneel in Rock Pose. Reach back and take hold of your heels. Using the abdominal muscles, arch the body up, with the arms straight. The chest lifts upward, and the head drops back. Press the hips forward to steady the pose. Breathe deeply or use Breath of Fire for 1 to 2 minutes.

◄ *In addition to bringing great flexibility to the spine, Camel Pose adjusts the navel point and relieves the stomach from the effects of overeating. Regular practice gives control over hunger and thirst. This pose also stretches the thigh muscles, which is said to control the calcium-magnesium balance in the body—necessary for both physical and mental well-being.*

1 **Frog Pose** Stand up with the heels close together and the feet spread outward. Squat down with the buttocks close to the heels, and the fingers on the floor, about a foot in front of the feet. The arms are between the knees, and the upper body is as straight as possible.

2 Inhale and straighten the legs, bringing the head close to the knees. Exhale and return to the original position. Try to keep the heels slightly off the ground the entire time. Continue for 15 to 26 repetitions, counting 1 inhale and 1 exhale as 1 repetition. Gradually increase the amount to a maximum of 108 repetitions. Relax for 2 to 5 minutes.

▲ *Frog Pose stimulates the energy of the first three chakras, associated with elimination, creativity, sexuality, and personal health and will. It then moves and circulates the energy to the heart and higher centers.*

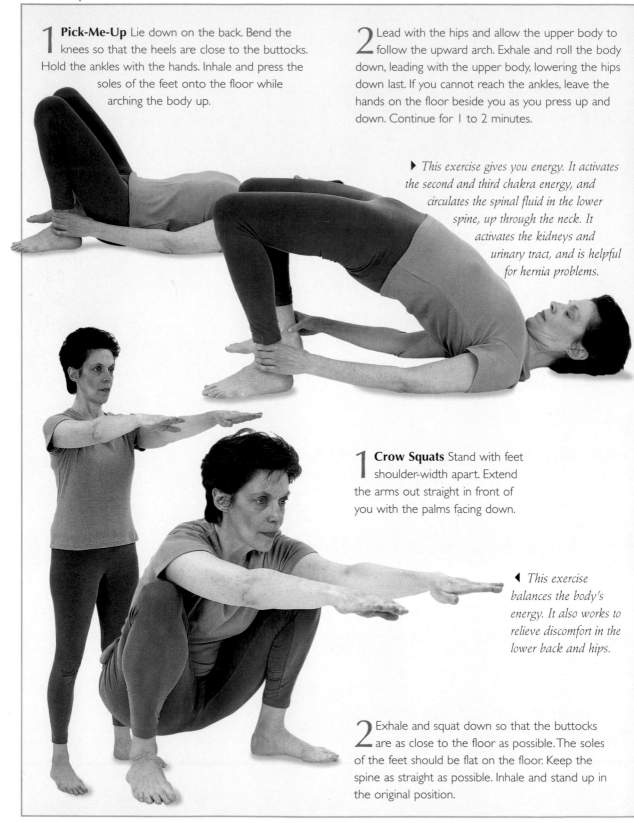

1 **Pick-Me-Up** Lie down on the back. Bend the knees so that the heels are close to the buttocks. Hold the ankles with the hands. Inhale and press the soles of the feet onto the floor while arching the body up.

2 Lead with the hips and allow the upper body to follow the upward arch. Exhale and roll the body down, leading with the upper body, lowering the hips down last. If you cannot reach the ankles, leave the hands on the floor beside you as you press up and down. Continue for 1 to 2 minutes.

▶ *This exercise gives you energy. It activates the second and third chakra energy, and circulates the spinal fluid in the lower spine, up through the neck. It activates the kidneys and urinary tract, and is helpful for hernia problems.*

1 **Crow Squats** Stand with feet shoulder-width apart. Extend the arms out straight in front of you with the palms facing down.

◀ *This exercise balances the body's energy. It also works to relieve discomfort in the lower back and hips.*

2 Exhale and squat down so that the buttocks are as close to the floor as possible. The soles of the feet should be flat on the floor. Keep the spine as straight as possible. Inhale and stand up in the original position.

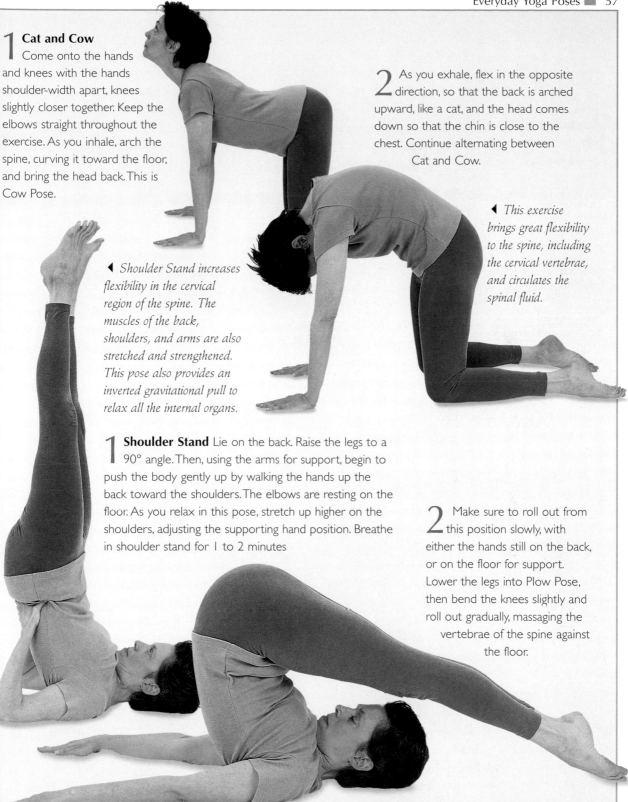

1 Cat and Cow
Come onto the hands and knees with the hands shoulder-width apart, knees slightly closer together. Keep the elbows straight throughout the exercise. As you inhale, arch the spine, curving it toward the floor, and bring the head back. This is Cow Pose.

2 As you exhale, flex in the opposite direction, so that the back is arched upward, like a cat, and the head comes down so that the chin is close to the chest. Continue alternating between Cat and Cow.

◀ *This exercise brings great flexibility to the spine, including the cervical vertebrae, and circulates the spinal fluid.*

◀ *Shoulder Stand increases flexibility in the cervical region of the spine. The muscles of the back, shoulders, and arms are also stretched and strengthened. This pose also provides an inverted gravitational pull to relax all the internal organs.*

1 Shoulder Stand Lie on the back. Raise the legs to a 90° angle. Then, using the arms for support, begin to push the body gently up by walking the hands up the back toward the shoulders. The elbows are resting on the floor. As you relax in this pose, stretch up higher on the shoulders, adjusting the supporting hand position. Breathe in shoulder stand for 1 to 2 minutes

2 Make sure to roll out from this position slowly, with either the hands still on the back, or on the floor for support. Lower the legs into Plow Pose, then bend the knees slightly and roll out gradually, massaging the vertebrae of the spine against the floor.

1 Plow Pose Lie down on the back. Bring the legs over
the head, supporting the body with the hands in the same
manner as in Shoulder Stand. Bring the legs straight out behind
you. If you can, place the balls of the feet on
the floor with the heels stretched away
from you. You can press the feet against a
wall if they do not reach the floor. Rest
the arms down on the floor with the
palms facing downward and flat.
Continue to hold this pose for 1 to 2
minutes. When finished, roll out in
the same manner
described
in Shoulder
Stand.

▼ *Plow Pose increases flexibility in the
cervical region of the spine. The muscles
of the back, shoulders, and arms are also
stretched and strengthened. Plow Pose
circulates kundalini energy and integrates
it into the entire body system, creating
stable and long-lasting effects.*

VARIATION

Plow Spread While in Plow Pose, spread
the legs apart, then inhale and lift up into a
spread Shoulder Stand. Exhale the legs back
down into Plow Spread and continue the
movement for 1 to 2 minutes.

1 Archer Pose Stand with the left leg
placed in front of you, pointing
forward, and the right leg placed in back
of you, pointing outward at a 45° angle
to the front foot. Straddle the legs
about 2½ feet apart. Raise the left
arm straight in front, parallel to
the ground, and make a fist as if
grasping a bow.

2 The right arm is pulled back as if pulling a
bowstring back to the shoulder. The right
forearm is parallel to the ground, and the hand is
in a fist. Both wrists form a straight line with the
arm. Bend the left knee and lean into it so that
you cannot see the right foot. Without leaning
forward, put 70 percent of your weight on the
front leg. Face forward and fix the eyes above
the fist, on the horizon. After holding 1 to 2
minutes, switch legs.

▲ *Archer Pose generates
fearlessness. It also balances
and strengthens the nervous
system.*

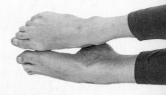

Triangle Pose

In a standing position, place the soles of the feet about 10 inches apart. Bend over and place the hands on the floor, shoulder-width apart. Keep the legs and arms straight. Your body forms a triangle with the buttocks at the highest point. The head is in line with the body.

▶ Triangle Pose aids in digestion, strengthens the entire nervous system, releases pent-up emotions, and relaxes the major muscle groups of the body.

Bundle Roll

Lie on the back with the arms pressed tightly against the sides, and the legs straight and pressed tightly together. Keeping the body straight, begin rolling sideways over and over, a few times one way, then back the other way. Do not bend anywhere. Use the power of your muscles to rock side to side until you have the momentum to roll over.

▼ Bundle Roll stimulates the entire body. It balances the electromagnetic field and massages the muscles.

CHAPTER 4

KUNDALINI YOGA KRIYAS

"You are spiritual beings here for a human experience."
–*Yogi Bhajan*

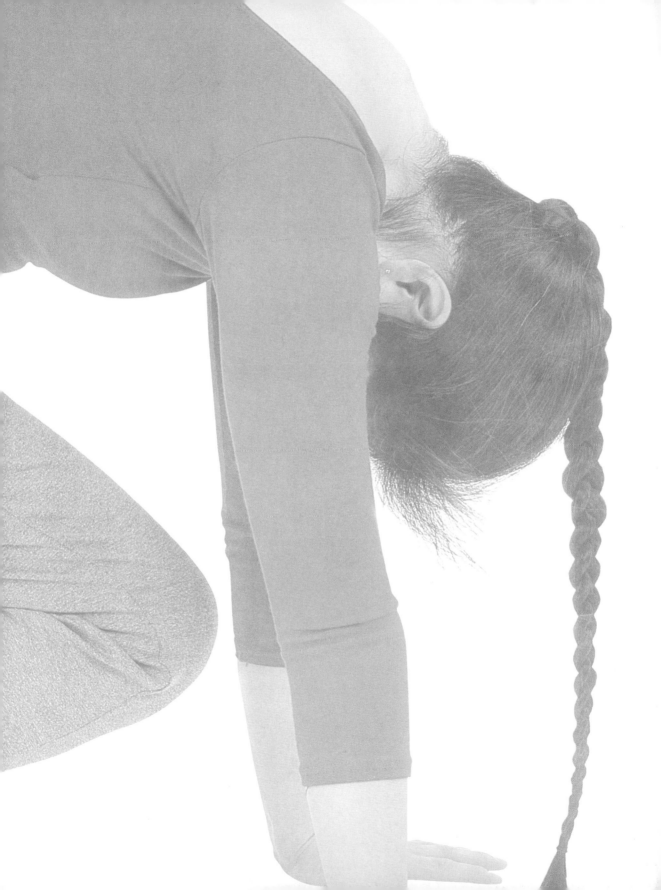

SELF-ADJUSTMENT OF
THE SPINE

Always make sure to warm up and stretch out your body before doing any set of exercises. This is especially true if you have back problems. The following kriya specifically works on creating a flexible, well-adjusted spine, surrounded by relaxed muscles.

▶ *Ideally, the heel of the raised foot should be resting on pelvic bone. There will be pressure at the base of the spine, and all the vertebrae will be automatically adjusted.*

1 Tree Pose Come into a standing position. Raise the left leg and place the heel of the foot against the pubic bone. The sole of the foot faces slightly upward, and the toes point toward the right hip. If this is too difficult, place the sole of the foot along the inside of the upper thigh with the heel close to the groin, and the toes pointing downward. Bring the palms together with the thumbs pressed into the chest at the heart center. This is called prayer pose.

Open the eyes and find a point of focus in the distance. Keep your gaze locked. This helps you to steady yourself in this pose. Raise the arms up overhead, hands remaining in prayer pose. Gently press the bent knee backward to straighten the spine further. Keep a constant upward pull and breathe long and deep. Remain in Tree Pose for 1 to 2 minutes. Then switch legs.

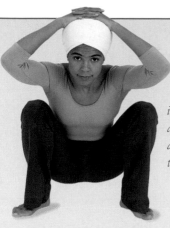

◀ *The angle of the back in this exercise allows the discs of the lower spine to adjust and balance themselves.*

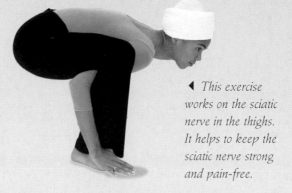

◀ *This exercise works on the sciatic nerve in the thighs. It helps to keep the sciatic nerve strong and pain-free.*

2 **Crow Squats** Stand up straight with your heels close together and your toes pointing slightly outward. Interlace your fingers and place the palms on top of your head. Bend the knees and lower the torso all the way down, keeping the heels on the ground if possible. Continue for 2-3 minutes.

3 **Buttocks Bounce** With legs shoulder-width apart, bend the knees into a semi-squat with the back parallel to the ground. The hands reach to the inside of the legs and firmly grasp the tops of the feet. Keep the head facing forward as you bounce the lower back and buttocks up and down 11 times, inhaling up and exhaling down. Use short, powerful breaths. Stand up and breathe normally for 5 seconds, then resume bouncing another 11 times. Continue the pattern for 2-3 mintues, then relax for 30 seconds, sitting in Easy Pose.

◀ *This exercise is very helpful in correcting the musculoskeletal system of the neck.*

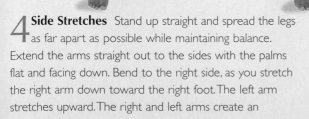

4 **Side Stretches** Stand up straight and spread the legs as far apart as possible while maintaining balance. Extend the arms straight out to the sides with the palms flat and facing down. Bend to the right side, as you stretch the right arm down toward the right foot. The left arm stretches upward. The right and left arms create an unbroken line. Hold the stretched position for 10 seconds. Then slowly and smoothly switch so that the left hand is touching the left foot without stopping in between. Keep the arms out straight from the shoulders in an unbroken line throughout the exercise. Continue for 1 to 3 minutes. Inhale, exhale, and relax on your back for a few minutes.

KRIYA FOR
DISEASE RESISTANCE

To avoid persistent colds and illness, it is essential to keep digestion and elimination functioning well. Add to this a strong metabolic balance and lymphatic system, and you will have heartiness. This kriya builds disease resistance and promotes robust health.

THE IMMUNE SYSTEM'S DEFENSE AGAINST INFECTION

One of the main functions of the immune system is to help the body fight infection. The thymus gland produces T cells that destroy virus infected cells. The bone marrow produces B cells that release molecules called antibodies. Antibodies aid in the destruction

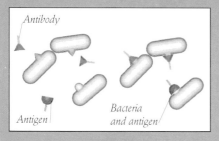

Antibody

Antigen

Bacteria and antigen

of disease-causing microorganisms by targeting specific molecules (antigens) on their surface. Bacteria are also killed by phagocytes

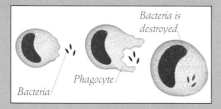

Bacteria is destroyed

Bacteria

Phagocyte

(eating cells). Phagocytes, led by a chemical trail, seek out, engulf, and destroy these foreign microorganisms.

1 Pumps Sit on your heels in rock pose. Stretch the arms straight overheard with the palms pressed together. Inhale and hold the breath. Pump the stomach by strongly drawing the navel in toward the spine and then relaxing it. Continue rhythmically until you must exhale. Exhale deeply. Inhale and begin again. Continue for 1 to 3 minutes, then inhale, exhale, and relax

▶ *This exercise stimulates digestion and the kundalini energy at the navel point (third chakra), which is the seat of physical health.*

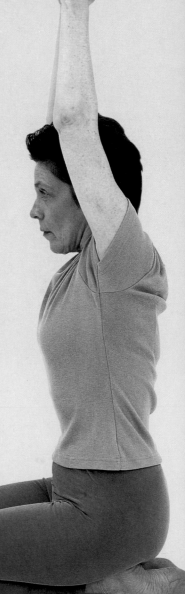

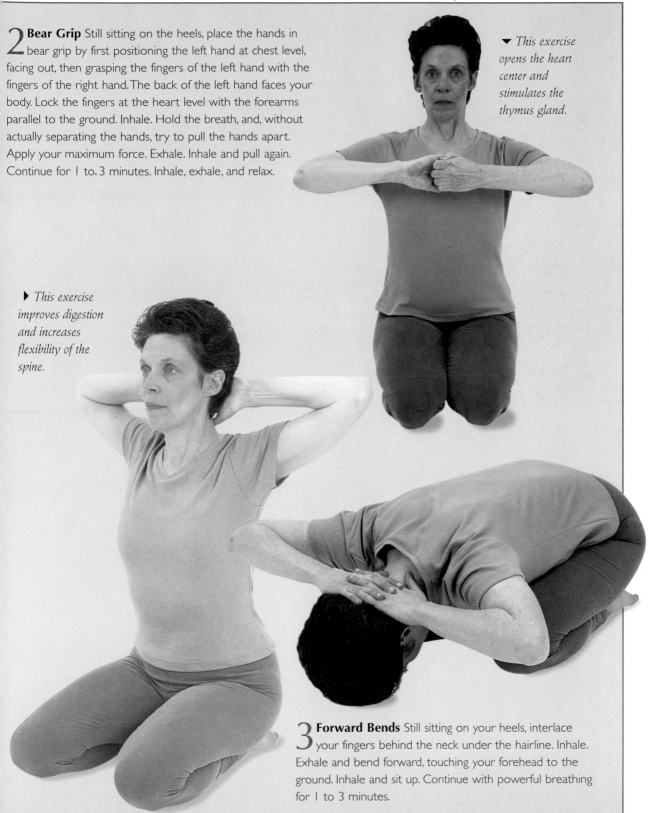

2 **Bear Grip** Still sitting on the heels, place the hands in bear grip by first positioning the left hand at chest level, facing out, then grasping the fingers of the left hand with the fingers of the right hand. The back of the left hand faces your body. Lock the fingers at the heart level with the forearms parallel to the ground. Inhale. Hold the breath, and, without actually separating the hands, try to pull the hands apart. Apply your maximum force. Exhale. Inhale and pull again. Continue for 1 to 3 minutes. Inhale, exhale, and relax.

▼ *This exercise opens the heart center and stimulates the thymus gland.*

▶ *This exercise improves digestion and increases flexibility of the spine.*

3 **Forward Bends** Still sitting on your heels, interlace your fingers behind the neck under the hairline. Inhale. Exhale and bend forward, touching your forehead to the ground. Inhale and sit up. Continue with powerful breathing for 1 to 3 minutes.

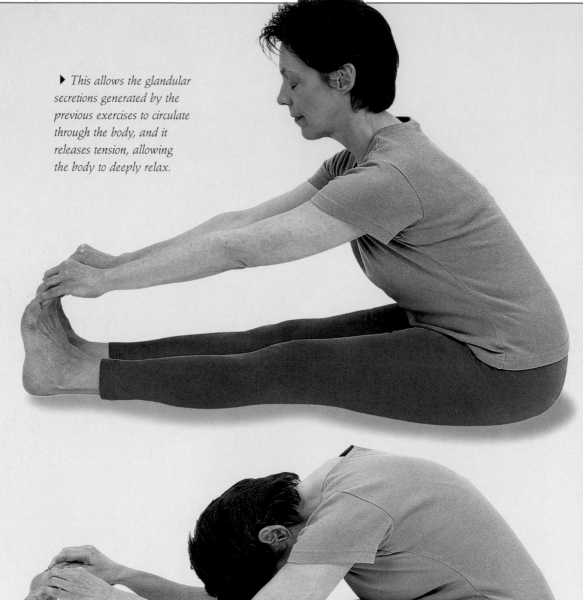

▶ *This allows the glandular secretions generated by the previous exercises to circulate through the body, and it releases tension, allowing the body to deeply relax.*

4 Leg Stretches Sit with the legs stretched out straight in front of you. Keep the legs flat on the ground as you reach forward, and, if possible, hold onto the toes as you inhale up. On the exhalation, stretch as far forward as possible. If you cannot reach your toes, reach your feet or ankles. Remain in this position, relaxing farther forward on each exhalation, for 1 to 3 minutes.

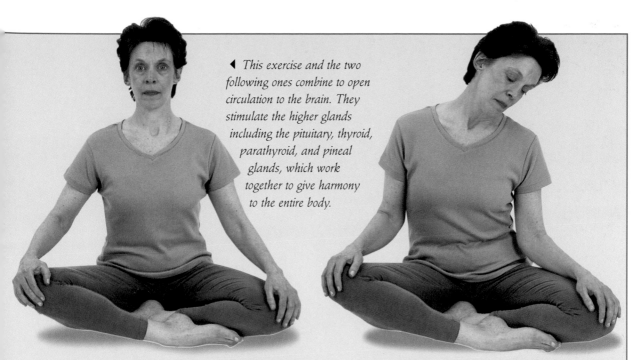

This exercise and the two following ones combine to open circulation to the brain. They stimulate the higher glands including the pituitary, thyroid, parathyroid, and pineal glands, which work together to give harmony to the entire body.

5 Neck Rolls Sit in Easy Pose. Begin by rolling the neck clockwise in a circular motion. Bring the right ear toward the shoulder as you inhale, then allow the head to roll toward the back. Exhale as the head comes around to the left. Continue for 1 to 2 minutes, then reverse the direction and continue for 1 to 2 minutes more.

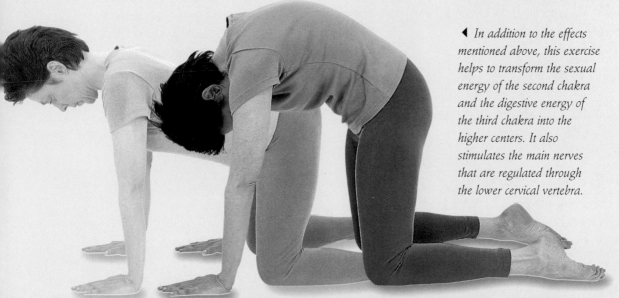

In addition to the effects mentioned above, this exercise helps to transform the sexual energy of the second chakra and the digestive energy of the third chakra into the higher centers. It also stimulates the main nerves that are regulated through the lower cervical vertebra.

6 Spine flex on Hands and Knees Kneel on the hands and knees with the hands shoulder-width apart, knees slightly closer together. The back is straight and parallel to the floor. As you inhale, arch the spine, curving it toward the floor. As you exhale, flex in the opposite direction, so that the back is arched upward.

This is the same as Cat and Cow Pose except that you keep the head down and relaxed throughout the exercise. Continue with a rhythmic breath for 1 to 3 minutes. Gradually increase your speed as you feel the spine becoming more flexible.

7 **Alternate Shoulder Shrugs** Sit on
your heels. Keeping the head still and
the chin slightly tucked, alternately shrug
each shoulder as high as possible. On the
inhalation, the left shoulder comes up
and the right goes down. On the
exhalation, the right comes up and the
left goes down. Continue rhythmically
with powerful breathing for 1 to 3
minutes. Inhale, raising both
shoulders. Exhale
and relax.

8 **Relaxation** Deeply
relax, lying on your
back with your arms at
your sides, palms facing
up, for 5 to 7 minutes.

9. **Triangle Pose:** Stand up. Bring the feet 6
inches apart. Bend over and place the
hands on the floor, around 2 feet apart. Keep
the legs and arms straight. Your body will form
a triangle with the buttocks at the highest
point. The head is in line with the body. Hold
this position for 2-5 minutes, breathing
normally. Then inhale, exhale, and slowly
come out of the position and relax.

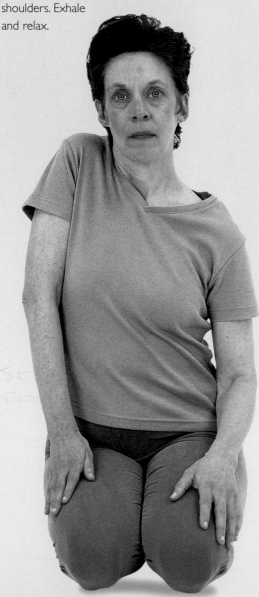

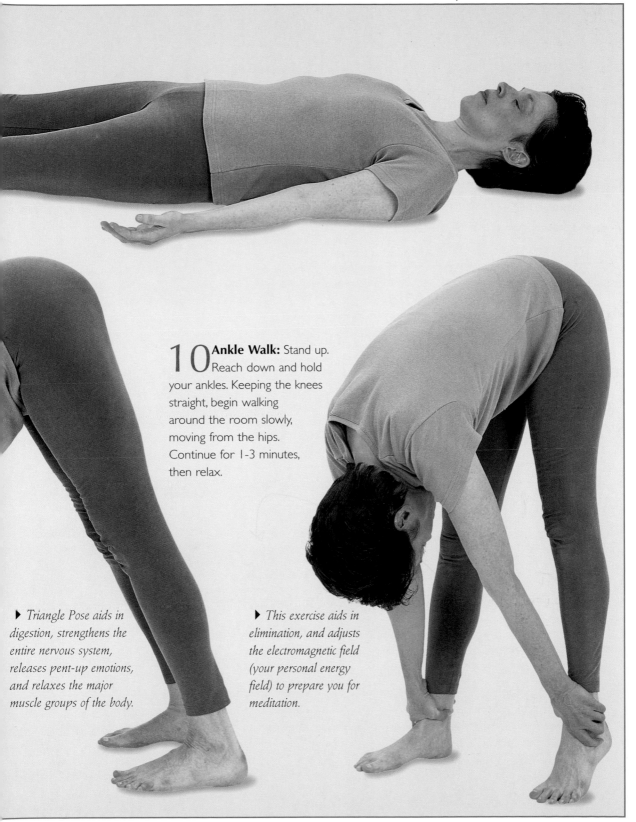

10 Ankle Walk: Stand up. Reach down and hold your ankles. Keeping the knees straight, begin walking around the room slowly, moving from the hips. Continue for 1-3 minutes, then relax.

▶ *Triangle Pose aids in digestion, strengthens the entire nervous system, releases pent-up emotions, and relaxes the major muscle groups of the body.*

▶ *This exercise aids in elimination, and adjusts the electromagnetic field (your personal energy field) to prepare you for meditation.*

TO MASTER
YOUR DOMAIN

To master your domain, you act from the center of your being, your command center. Mentally, this means that you are able to hold and project a thought, an idea, into reality. In the physical body, you are able to circulate blood from the core to all the outlying limbs and glands. This kriya gives you command in both the mental and physical realms. Followed by meditation, this kriya gives the spirit of a saint and the fearlessness of a warrior.

▶ *This and the following exercise strengthen the navel center, which is the seat of your personal power. The powerful breathing pattern quickens the effects of the exercises.*

SEAT OF POWER

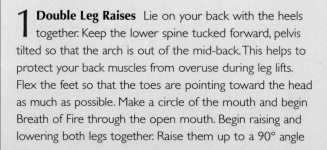

1 Double Leg Raises Lie on your back with the heels together. Keep the lower spine tucked forward, pelvis tilted so that the arch is out of the mid-back. This helps to protect your back muscles from overuse during leg lifts. Flex the feet so that the toes are pointing toward the head as much as possible. Make a circle of the mouth and begin Breath of Fire through the open mouth. Begin raising and lowering both legs together. Raise them up to a 90° angle and back down again, keeping the legs straight and the feet flexed. Hands are on the floor by the sides, or if necessary, under the buttocks for lower spine support. Continue to move the legs up and down with Breath of Fire through the circled mouth for 2 to 5 minutes. Then inhale and hold your legs up briefly. Slowly lower your legs to the ground as you exhale. Rest for 30 seconds, breathing long and light.

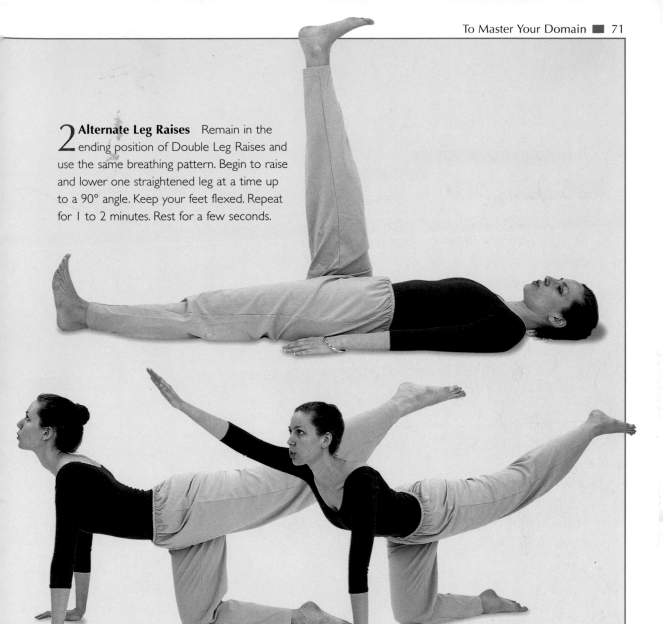

2 Alternate Leg Raises Remain in the ending position of Double Leg Raises and use the same breathing pattern. Begin to raise and lower one straightened leg at a time up to a 90° angle. Keep your feet flexed. Repeat for 1 to 2 minutes. Rest for a few seconds.

3 Extended Cow Pose #1 Kneel on the hands and knees with the back straight and parallel to the floor. The head is back, chin pointing toward the ceiling, and spine slightly arched downward, like a cow. Using the same breathing pattern as in the previous two exercises, begin to raise and lower alternate legs, extending them as high as possible without twisting the pelvis. Stay in Cow Pose with the head up and the spine slightly arched downward as you continue for 2 to 4 minutes. Inhale deeply and stretch up, then relax.

4 Extended Cow Pose #2 Remain in the ending position of Extended Cow Pose #1. The breath and movement are the same, except that you will raise opposite arms and legs at the same time. First the right leg and left arm extend up and out, then the left leg and right arm. Keep the eyes slightly open for balance. Continue for 1 to 2 minutes. Inhale deeply, stretching, then relax. Sit quietly on your heels for 30 seconds and breathe. Circulate the internal energy.

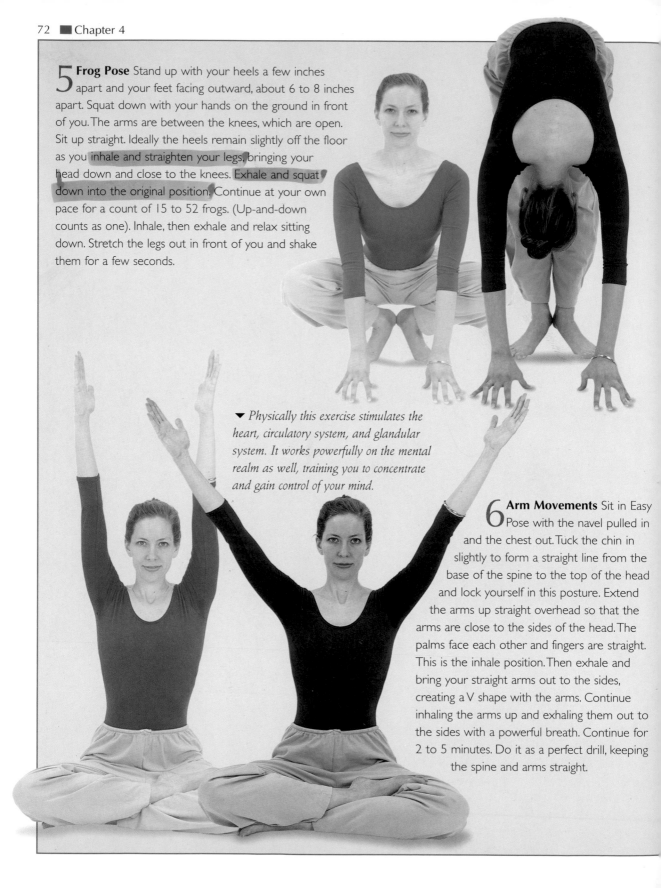

5 Frog Pose Stand up with your heels a few inches apart and your feet facing outward, about 6 to 8 inches apart. Squat down with your hands on the ground in front of you. The arms are between the knees, which are open. Sit up straight. Ideally the heels remain slightly off the floor as you inhale and straighten your legs, bringing your head down and close to the knees. Exhale and squat down into the original position. Continue at your own pace for a count of 15 to 52 frogs. (Up-and-down counts as one). Inhale, then exhale and relax sitting down. Stretch the legs out in front of you and shake them for a few seconds.

▼ *Physically this exercise stimulates the heart, circulatory system, and glandular system. It works powerfully on the mental realm as well, training you to concentrate and gain control of your mind.*

6 Arm Movements Sit in Easy Pose with the navel pulled in and the chest out. Tuck the chin in slightly to form a straight line from the base of the spine to the top of the head and lock yourself in this posture. Extend the arms up straight overhead so that the arms are close to the sides of the head. The palms face each other and fingers are straight. This is the inhale position. Then exhale and bring your straight arms out to the sides, creating a V shape with the arms. Continue inhaling the arms up and exhaling them out to the sides with a powerful breath. Continue for 2 to 5 minutes. Do it as a perfect drill, keeping the spine and arms straight.

7 Meditate Remain in Easy Pose. Breathe long and deep and meditate for 2 to 5 minutes. If you like, have some beautiful, uplifting music playing for this and the following exercise. (See "Resources" for companion CD.)

8 Heart-cross Lie down on your back, legs still folded and crossed at the ankles. Cross your hands over your heart. Relax in this position and breathe long and light for a few minutes.

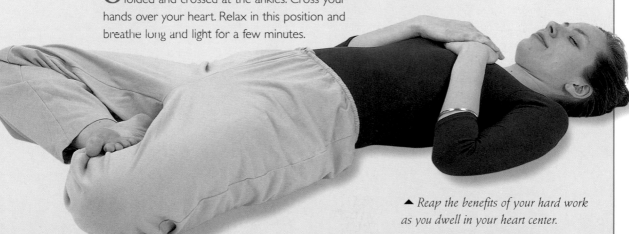

▲ *Reap the benefits of your hard work as you dwell in your heart center.*

THE ESSENCE OF SELF

This series of exercises guides the pranic life force through the body to the heart center, "opening" the heart so that you can give and receive love without fear, anger, or resentment. This state of compassion is the essence of self. When feeling weighted down by the scars and disappointments of life, this kriya will help you sense the broader reality of which you are a part. All possibilities open to you when you live from the essence of self. Physically, this kriya releases tension, strengthens digestion, and opens the lungs.

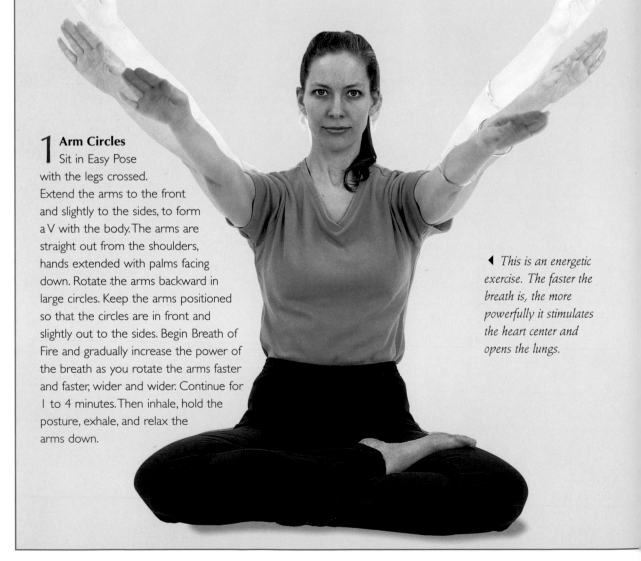

1 Arm Circles

Sit in Easy Pose with the legs crossed. Extend the arms to the front and slightly to the sides, to form a V with the body. The arms are straight out from the shoulders, hands extended with palms facing down. Rotate the arms backward in large circles. Keep the arms positioned so that the circles are in front and slightly out to the sides. Begin Breath of Fire and gradually increase the power of the breath as you rotate the arms faster and faster, wider and wider. Continue for 1 to 4 minutes. Then inhale, hold the posture, exhale, and relax the arms down.

◀ *This is an energetic exercise. The faster the breath is, the more powerfully it stimulates the heart center and opens the lungs.*

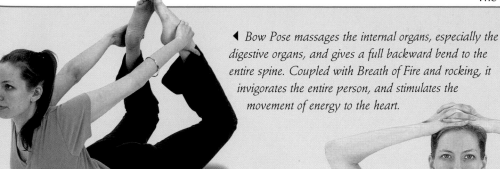

◀ *Bow Pose massages the internal organs, especially the digestive organs, and gives a full backward bend to the entire spine. Coupled with Breath of Fire and rocking, it invigorates the entire person, and stimulates the movement of energy to the heart.*

2 Rocking Bow

Lie on the stomach and assume Bow Pose: Reach back and take hold of the ankles, stretching up by creating a tension between the arms and legs. Rock back and forth from the shoulders to the knees, coordinating the motion with a powerful Breath of Fire, so powerful that it feels as though fire were coming from the nostrils. Continue for 1 minute. Then relax briefly.

◀ *Crow squats allow the pelvis to relax and open.*

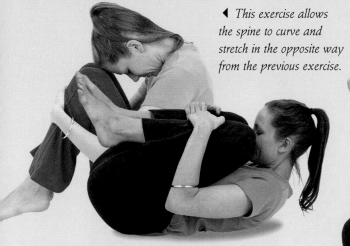

◀ *This exercise allows the spine to curve and stretch in the opposite way from the previous exercise.*

3 Rock on Spine

Lie on the back with the thighs clasped to the chest, forehead to the knees. Rock along the entire length of the spine in conjunction with Breath of Fire for 1 minute.

4 Crow Squats

Stand with feet 1 to 1½ feet apart. The feet face forward, turned slightly outward. Interlace the fingers in Venus Lock on top of the head. Exhale and crouch down so that the buttocks are as close to the floor as possible. Ideally, the feet remain flat on the floor. Keep the spine as straight as possible. Then inhale and return to the standing position. Continue for 26 squats.

5 Arm Circles

Repeat the first exercise of this kriya for 1 to 2 minutes.

6 Essence of Self Meditation Sitting in Easy Pose, cross the hands at the center of the chest, over the heart center. Close the eyes. Remain focused and meditate for 5 to 31 minutes. If available, meditate with or sing some divine, uplifting music. (See "Resources" for companion CD.)

◀ *Drop any self-limitations. Surrender the self to the Self. In this expanded awareness you will experience your essence.*

MOVEMENT RELAXATION

Rhythmic, unforced, graceful, and free movement relaxes the entire body and mind. It releases the tensions stored in the body from our everyday emotions. All emotional traumas leave their signature of tension in the body. If these areas are not relaxed, the built-up stress can lead to both physical and mental health imbalances.

1 Movement Stand straight with arms completely relaxed. Close the eyes. Notice any tension by mentally scanning the entire body. Allow the tension to release in each part. Consciously let it go. Next, begin to sway and move every part of the body. Dance, feeling the easy movement of each body area. If there is gentle rhythmic music of a high vibration available, it may be used as a background. Continue for 3 to 11 minutes, or as long as you like. (See "Resources" for music suggestions.)

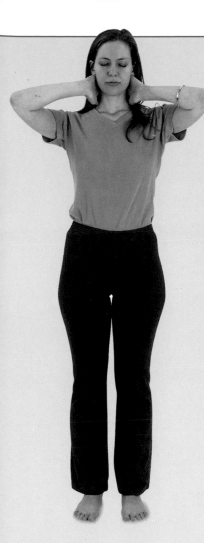

2 Touch Stand straight with the eyes still closed. With the hands, begin to lightly feel each part of the body without reservation. Every square inch must be touched. Feel sensitively with the palms of the hands. Bless yourself with your touch. Continue for 2 to 5 minutes.

▼ *The Forward and Backward Hangs strengthen the heart and circulatory system. If this system is weak, tissues in the extremities and joints may build up deposits that create illness.*

Feeling the entire body confirms the reality of the relaxation, is self-healing, and smooths the aura (surrounding energy field).

3 Forward Hang Lean forward with arms hanging completely relaxed. Keep the knees relaxed and unlocked. Allow every muscle in the body to relax. Let the breath be normal. Continue for 2 to 11 minutes.

4 Backward Hang Inhale and exhale deeply several times. Slowly straighten and, in a continuous motion, slowly lean back with arms hanging loosely down from shoulders. The breath is relaxed. Continue for 1 minute. Then slowly straighten and completely relax.

WAHE GURU
SUBTLE BODY KRIYA

This is an example of a meditative yoga kriya that uses mantra. Physically, the set is a total workout for the thyroid, pituitary, and pineal glands. It also works on the subtle body, that part of your being that understands beyond the obvious. When the subtle body is strong, you are calm and masterful.

In each of the first five exercises, the mantra used is *Wha* (use the lips to create the sound water makes as it pours from a bottle), a soft, almost inaudible *hay*, then *Guru* (g'roo, softly rolling the sound of the *r* off the roof of the mouth). *Wahe Guru* is the expression of indescribable ecstasy, of union with the Infinite.

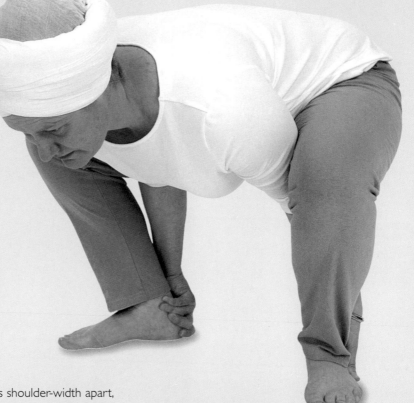

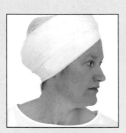

For the first 3 exercises in this set, the head turns left when chanting Wahe, *and right when chanting* Guru.

1 Chair Pose With the legs shoulder-width apart, bend the knees into a semi-squat with the back parallel to the ground. The hands grasp the heels firmly. Keep the spine straight throughout. The neck is in line with the spine and the head faces the floor. Turn the head to the left, so the chin comes over the left shoulder, and chant *Wahe*. Then turn the head to the right, with the chin coming over the right shoulder, and chant *Guru*. Alternate at a moderate pace to make a continuous sound current of *Wahe Guru, Wahe Guru, Wahe Guru*. Continue 1 to 3 minutes. Inhale, exhale, and relax the pose.

2 **Backward Lean** Stand up with the feet shoulder-width apart. Put the hands on the hips (where your back pants' pockets would be) and lean backwards. Keep the legs straight, with unlocked knees. Let the head fall back. Turn the head to the left with *Wahe*, to the right with *Guru*. The head moves in an arc. Continue for 1 to 3 minutes. Inhale, exhale, and relax.

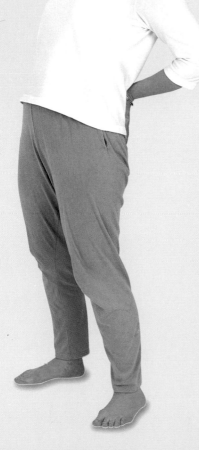

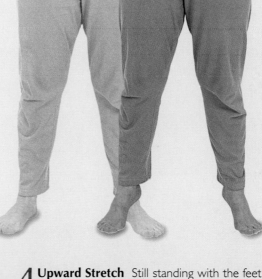

3 **Forward Lean** Stand with feet shoulder-width apart. Bend forward slightly, hands resting on the thighs, close to the knees. The spine is straight throughout. With the shoulders relaxed, stretch the neck outward and tilt the chin slightly upward. Turn the head to the left with *Wahe* and to the right with *Guru*. Continue for 1 to 3 minutes. Inhale, exhale, and relax.

4 **Upward Stretch** Still standing with the feet shoulder-width apart, stretch the arms straight overhead with the fingers spread apart. Keep a full upward stretch. As you chant *Wahe*, keep the feet flat on the ground. On *Guru*, rise up on the toes. Continue up and down for 1 to 3 minutes. Inhale, exhale, and relax.

5 **Sphinx** Sit on the heels. Place the palms flat on the floor just in front of the knees. The spine and arms are straight, looking like a sphinx. Stretch the neck out of the shoulders, which relax downward. In this position, chant *Wahe*. Then, still keeping the spine somewhat straight, bend forward, touching the forehead to the ground, and chant *Guru*. Continue for 1 to 3 minutes. Then inhale, exhale, and relax.

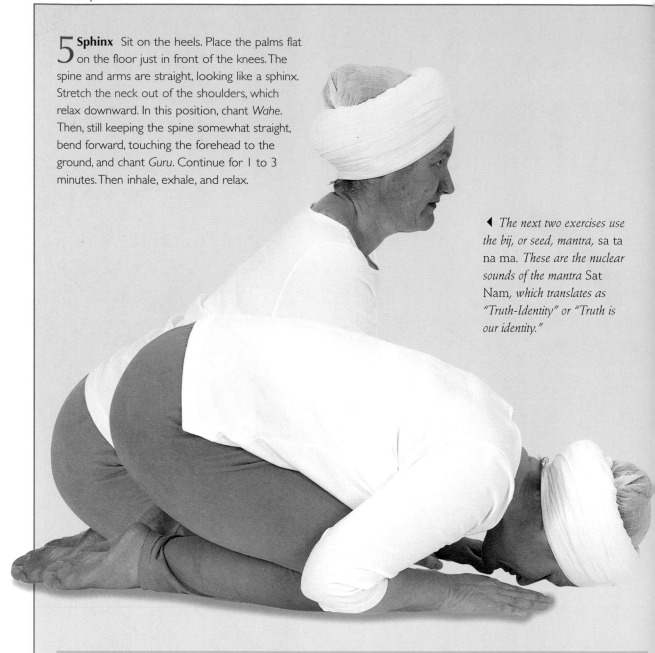

◀ *The next two exercises use the bij, or seed, mantra,* sa ta na ma. *These are the nuclear sounds of the mantra* Sat Nam, *which translates as "Truth-Identity" or "Truth is our identity."*

Gian Mudra

Gian Mudra increases wisdom. It uses the index finger, which is represented by the planet Jupiter–the planet of expansion. This mudra is used with most meditative postures.

To form passive *Gian Mudra*, put the tip of the thumb together with the tip of the index finger. This stimulates knowledge and wisdom within you. It also increases receptivity and calmness.

To form active *Gian Mudra*, curl the index finger under the thumb so that the fingernail is on the second joint of the thumb. This generates all of the same qualities as passive *Gian Mudra*, but with a more active, or projective energy.

6 Meditation Sit in Easy Pose with the spine straight. The hands are in *Gian Mudra*. Begin to whisper the bij mantra: *sa ta na ma*, using the musical notation below. Continue for 1 to 2 minutes, then chant loudly for 1 to 2 minutes more.

7 Spine Flex Immediately after meditation, sit on the heels with the palms on the thighs. Begin flexing the spine and chanting in a powerful whisper in the following way: As you arch the spine forward, chest out, chant *sa*; as you curve back, and shoulders come forward, chant *ta*. Again, arch forward for *na*, and back for *ma*. Continue for 1 to 3 minutes. Inhale, exhale, and relax on the back.

▶ *Meditation after this kriya brings the realization that we are channels for truth, and that to maintain grace in the most ungraceful moments is the true human worth.*

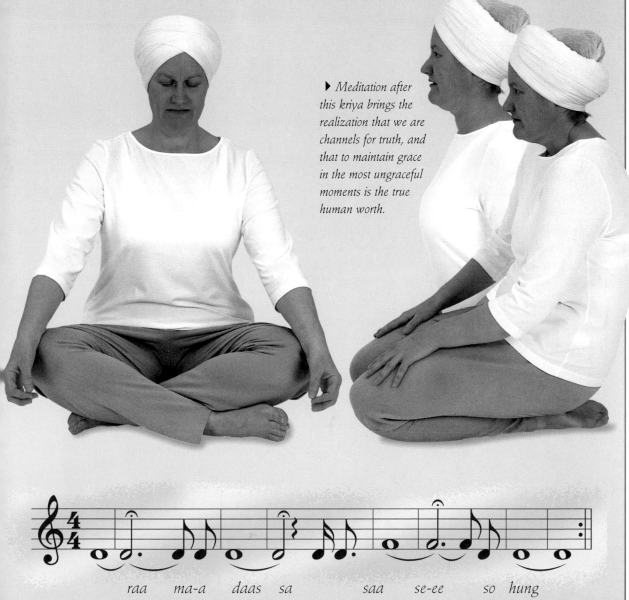

raa   ma-a   daas   sa   saa   se-ee   so   hung

KRIYA FOR
PELVIC BALANCE

When you move in balance and grace, you feel connected to the earth and ready to act. This experience is physical as well as mental. When the pelvis and the muscles that shape its posture are out of balance, many systems of the body will begin to show signs of stress. Exhaustion, low endurance, and lower back pain are common symptoms of this condition. This kriya is helpful for staying energetic and balanced, as well as for maintaining potency if practiced regularly.

With this, and any strenuous set of exercises, it is advisable to do warm-up exercises first. Beginners should approach these exercises slowly and carefully.

1 **Bridge Pose** Sit with the feet flat on the floor and shoulder-width apart. Place the hands on the floor behind you, fingers pointing away from the body. Lean back slightly. Raise the body, supporting it with straight arms and bent legs. The body from the knees to the shoulders forms a straight line that is parallel to the ground. Let the head fall back slightly. Apply the Root Lock (see page 35) as you hold the posture, breathing normally. Continue for 1 to 3 minutes. Then inhale, exhale, and relax down.

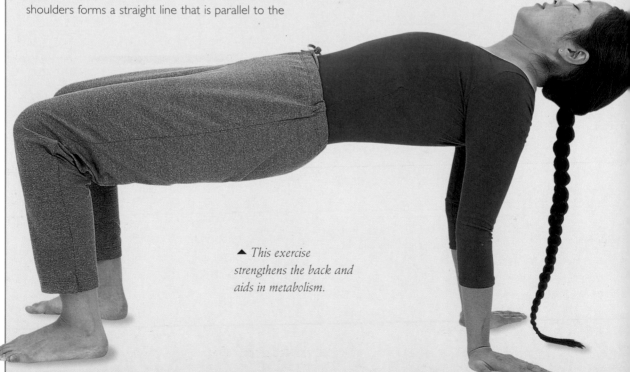

▲ *This exercise strengthens the back and aids in metabolism.*

A Preparatory Alternative to Wheel Pose

Bring ankles close to the buttocks. Hold the ankles and gently stretch the body up on the inhalation, leading with the hips. Exhale down, leading with the upper spine and bringing the hips down last. Repeat several times. Then hold the arched position, pressing the heels into the floor. Breathe long and deep or use Breath of Fire.

Using props such as a few large pillows or a body ball can help provide support to the arched back. Place the feet and hands on the floor as in Wheel Pose. Arch, stretch, and breathe long and deep or use Breath of Fire.

2 **Wheel Pose** Lie on the back. Bend the legs, with the soles of the feet pressed against the floor, close to the buttocks. Bending the elbows, place the palms of the hands on the floor above the shoulders with the fingers pointing back toward the shoulders. Keeping the feet and knees parallel, begin to carefully lift the body off the floor by pushing against the floor with the hands and feet. Lead with the hips, followed by the chest. The neck arches back as you straighten the elbows. The body forms one continuous arch from the heels to the hands. In this position begin Breath of Fire. Continue for 30 seconds to 3 minutes. Inhale deeply. Exhale as you slowly and carefully let yourself down and relax on your back.

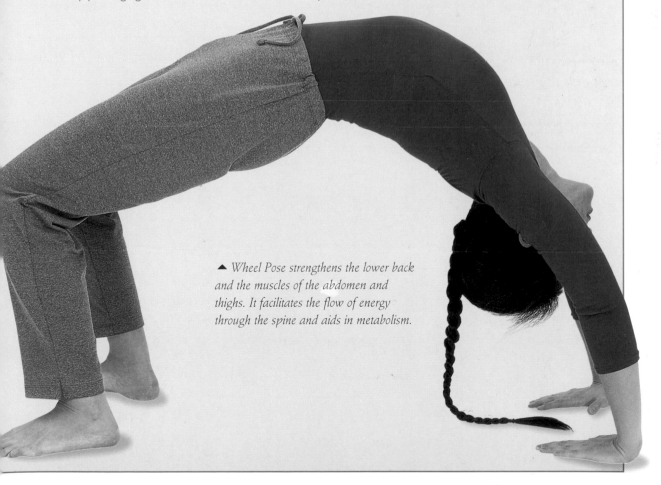

▲ *Wheel Pose strengthens the lower back and the muscles of the abdomen and thighs. It facilitates the flow of energy through the spine and aids in metabolism.*

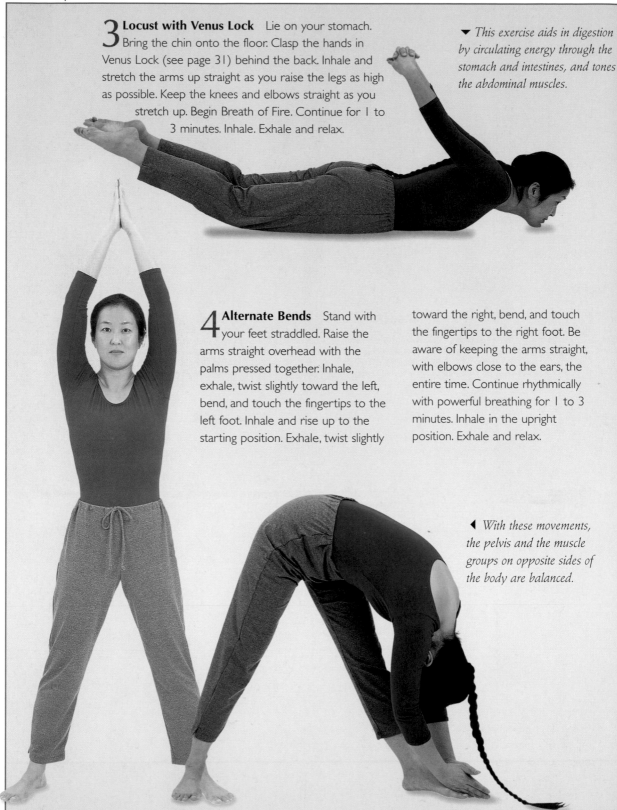

3 Locust with Venus Lock   Lie on your stomach. Bring the chin onto the floor. Clasp the hands in Venus Lock (see page 31) behind the back. Inhale and stretch the arms up straight as you raise the legs as high as possible. Keep the knees and elbows straight as you stretch up. Begin Breath of Fire. Continue for 1 to 3 minutes. Inhale. Exhale and relax.

▼ *This exercise aids in digestion by circulating energy through the stomach and intestines, and tones the abdominal muscles.*

4 Alternate Bends   Stand with your feet straddled. Raise the arms straight overhead with the palms pressed together. Inhale, exhale, twist slightly toward the left, bend, and touch the fingertips to the left foot. Inhale and rise up to the starting position. Exhale, twist slightly toward the right, bend, and touch the fingertips to the right foot. Be aware of keeping the arms straight, with elbows close to the ears, the entire time. Continue rhythmically with powerful breathing for 1 to 3 minutes. Inhale in the upright position. Exhale and relax.

◀ *With these movements, the pelvis and the muscle groups on opposite sides of the body are balanced.*

▶ *This exercise helps to channel second chakra (creative/sexual) energy and maintain potency. Pressing the top of the big toe stimulates the pituitary gland.*

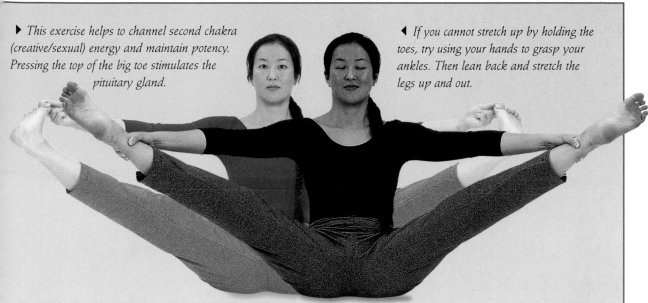

◀ *If you cannot stretch up by holding the toes, try using your hands to grasp your ankles. Then lean back and stretch the legs up and out.*

5 Kundalini Lotus Sit with the soles of the feet together. Wrap the first finger of each hand around the big toes and press the top of the toes with the thumbs. Lean back slightly and stretch the legs up to a 60-degree angle from the ground. The legs are spread, the knees straight. Balance on the buttocks. To maintain your balance, keep the eyes open and focus on a point some distance from you. Begin Breath of Fire. Continue for 1 to 3 minutes. Inhale. Exhale and relax.

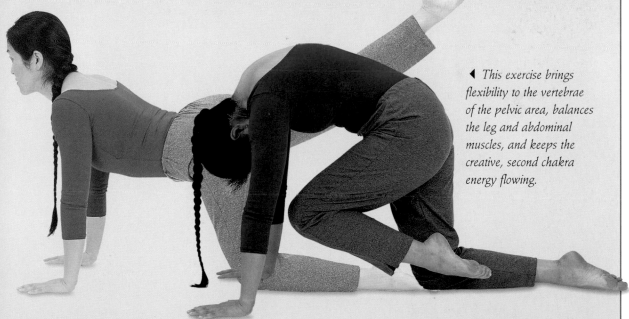

◀ *This exercise brings flexibility to the vertebrae of the pelvic area, balances the leg and abdominal muscles, and keeps the creative, second chakra energy flowing.*

6 Leg Swings Come into Cow Pose, supporting the body on the hands and knees, both shoulder-width apart. Inhale and stretch the head up and arch the spine. Meanwhile, lift the right leg straight up behind you, keeping the hip straight. Exhale and curve the spine, bringing the knee and forehead together. The spine arches and curves as you continue with the right leg for 1 to 3 minutes. Then inhale and exhale. Repeat the exercise using the left leg for 1 to 3 minutes. Then inhale, exhale, and deeply relax on your back for 5 minutes or more.

BECOMING
LIKE ANGELS

This is a powerfully transforming kriya that will give you the health and internal energy to live from your angelic nature.

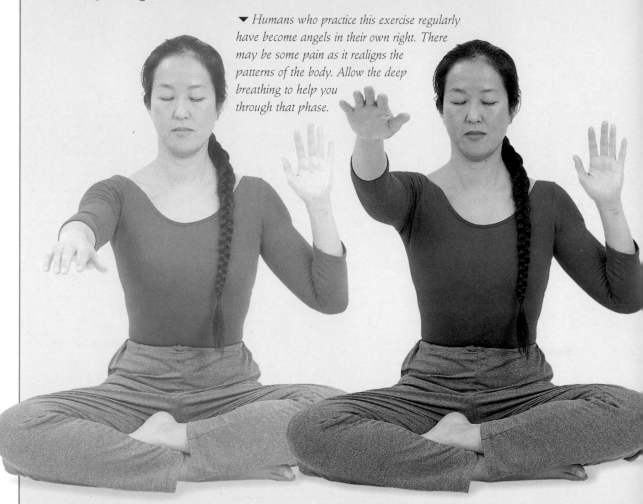

▼ *Humans who practice this exercise regularly have become angels in their own right. There may be some pain as it realigns the patterns of the body. Allow the deep breathing to help you through that phase.*

1 Patting Air Sit in Easy Pose. Stretch the right arm forward with the palm facing down. The left elbow is bent and the upper arm is close to the side of the body. The left palm is flat, facing forward with fingers straight (as though taking an oath). Move the right arm as though patting the air. Go up about 30 degrees above horizontal and back down to parallel to the floor. Keep the arm straight, move from the shoulder, and pat at a speed of 30 times per minute. Close your eyes. Inhale through the nose and exhale through the mouth. Breathe slowly, heavily, and deeply. Continue for 3 to 6 minutes.

2 Switch Sides Change hands and repeat the first exercise in this kriya for 2 to 3 minutes.

3 Shoulder Roll Relax and roll your shoulders. Continue loosening the shoulders for 1 to 2 minutes.

4 Balance Bend both elbows, keeping the upper arms close to the ribs. The wrists are bent and the palms face upward. The fingers point away from the body at a diagonal. The eyes focus on the tip of the nose in a steady, soft gaze. Inhale through the nose and exhale through the mouth as fast and powerfully as you can. Hold your arms and shoulders in perfect balance. There will be tremendous pressure on the chest. Continue for 3 to 5½ minutes.

▶ *This exercise works on eliminating chronic illness.*

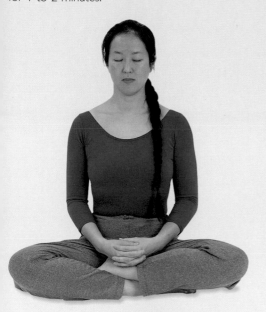

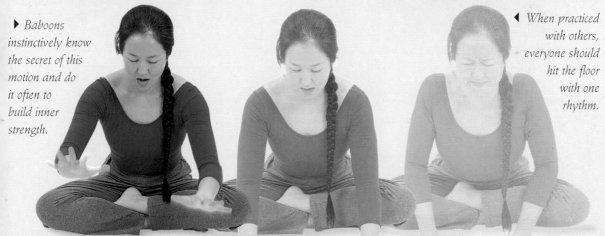

▶ *Baboons instinctively know the secret of this motion and do it often to build inner strength.*

◀ *When practiced with others, everyone should hit the floor with one rhythm.*

5 Clap the ground Rhythmically hit the ground in front of you with both hands at the same time, keeping the spine fairly straight. As you hit the ground, chant *Har* (The Infinite One), using only the tip of the tongue on the roof of the mouth as you roll the *r* sound. Use the power of the navel point to chant, and hit powerfully. Go for 3 to 6½ minutes. Then inhale and hold the breath 15 to 20 seconds while you tense all your muscles and press the hands against the ground with the entire weight of the body. Exhale explosively through the mouth. Repeat this sequence 2 more times.

6 Stretch and Move Take 2 minutes to recover from the powerful effects of this kriya. Do not meditate or be silent at this time. Stretch, walk around, and talk to ground yourself.

NABHI KRIYA
FOR THE NAVEL CENTER

This set focuses on developing the strength of the navel (or *Nabhi*) center. The navel center is the seat of your physical well-being. In our prenatal stage, we were fed at the navel point. It was our lifeline and major center of energy. As adults, we still have that navel/lifeline connection, but it is an energetic connection to the infinite source.

On the psychological level, a strong, balanced navel chakra gives the power to maintain a course of action. It gives the ability to break habits and create new ones. This set helps release blocks in the navel center, allowing the energy to be transformed to the higher centers. Practicing Nabhi Kriya before meditating helps sustain the effect of meditation and integrate it into the personality.

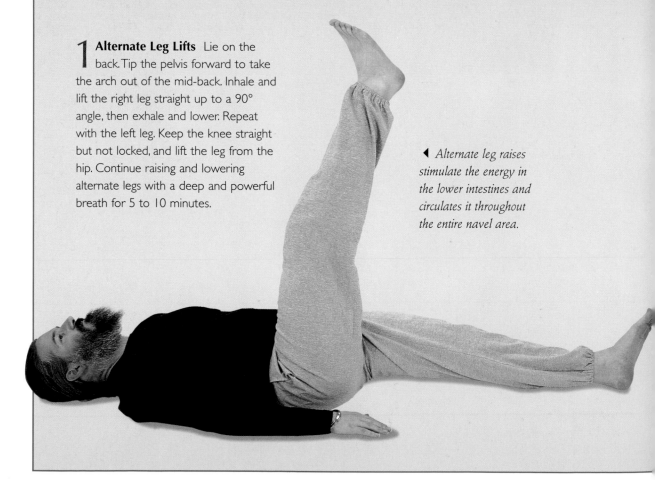

1 **Alternate Leg Lifts** Lie on the back. Tip the pelvis forward to take the arch out of the mid-back. Inhale and lift the right leg straight up to a 90° angle, then exhale and lower. Repeat with the left leg. Keep the knee straight but not locked, and lift the leg from the hip. Continue raising and lowering alternate legs with a deep and powerful breath for 5 to 10 minutes.

◀ *Alternate leg raises stimulate the energy in the lower intestines and circulates it throughout the entire navel area.*

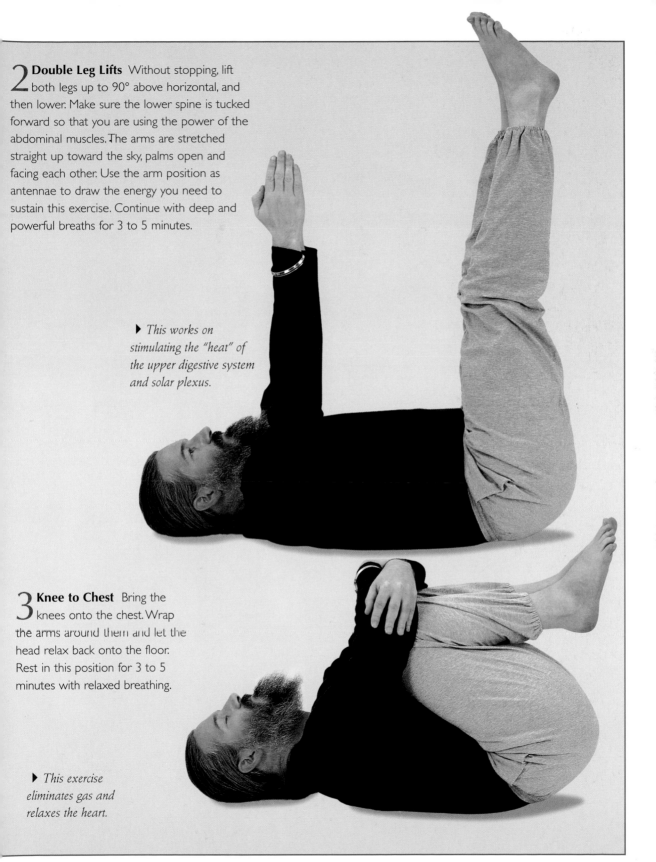

2 Double Leg Lifts Without stopping, lift both legs up to 90° above horizontal, and then lower. Make sure the lower spine is tucked forward so that you are using the power of the abdominal muscles. The arms are stretched straight up toward the sky, palms open and facing each other. Use the arm position as antennae to draw the energy you need to sustain this exercise. Continue with deep and powerful breaths for 3 to 5 minutes.

▶ *This works on stimulating the "heat" of the upper digestive system and solar plexus.*

3 Knee to Chest Bring the knees onto the chest. Wrap the arms around them and let the head relax back onto the floor. Rest in this position for 3 to 5 minutes with relaxed breathing.

▶ *This exercise eliminates gas and relaxes the heart.*

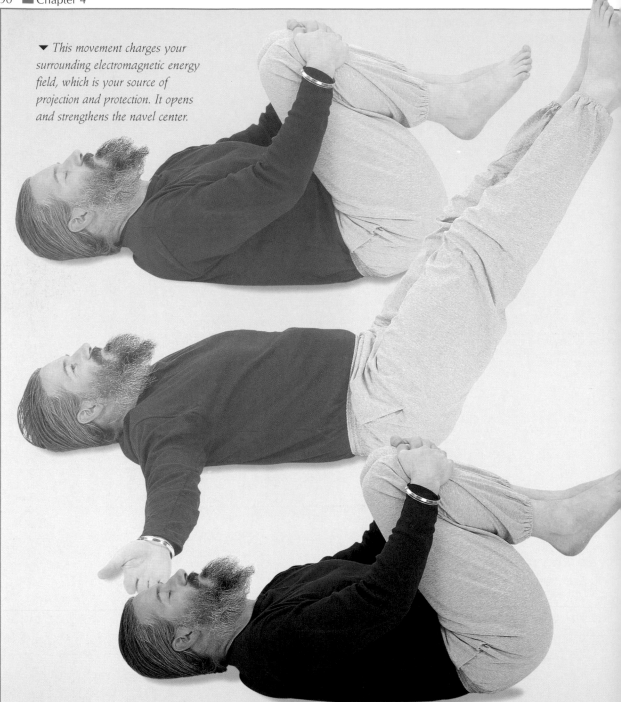

▼ *This movement charges your surrounding electromagnetic energy field, which is your source of projection and protection. It opens and strengthens the navel center.*

4 **Contract/Extend** Starting with the ending position of Knees to Chest, inhale and open the arms straight out to the sides and onto the ground. At the same time extend the legs straight out to a 60° angle from the ground (almost ⅔ of the way to perpendicular). On the exhalation, return to the original position with the arms wrapped around the bent legs. On the extension, lead with the pointed toes. Use the abdominal muscles to control the gradual extension and straightening of the legs. Continue for 7 to 15 minutes.

5 Rapid Leg Raises Continue to lie on the back. Bring the left knee to the chest. Hold it there with both hands wrapped around. Begin rapidly lifting the right leg up to a 90° angle, and back down to the floor. Keep the knee straight throughout and lift the leg from the hip. Breathe powerfully, inhaling as the leg goes up, exhaling as it moves down. Continue for 1 minute, then switch to the left leg. Repeat with the left leg. After 1 minute, switch legs again and repeat the exercise for 1 more minute on each leg.

▶ *This raises the kundalini energy and circulates it throughout the entire spine, spinal fluid, and into the aura.*

▼ *This exercise sets the hips and lower spine.*

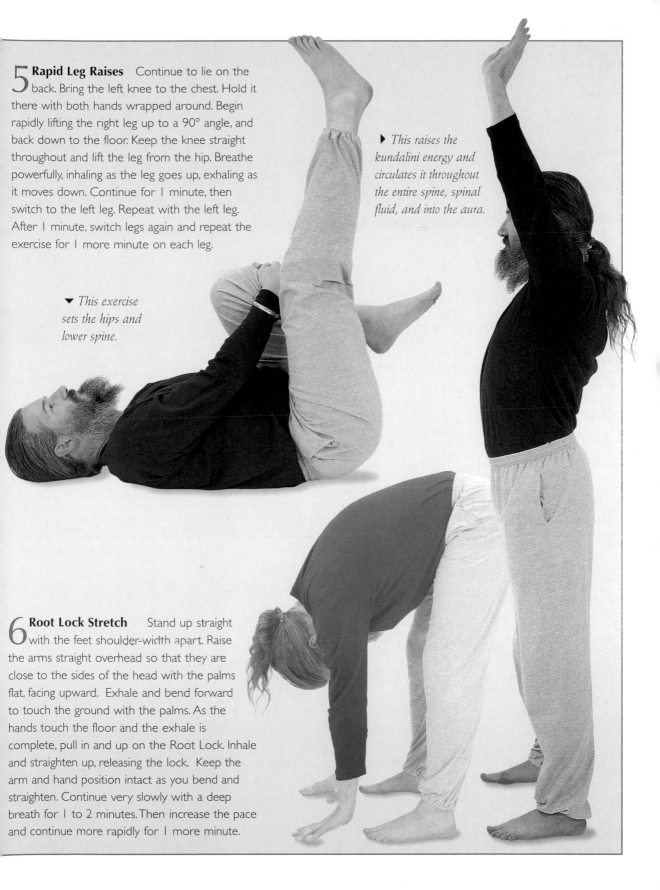

6 Root Lock Stretch Stand up straight with the feet shoulder-width apart. Raise the arms straight overhead so that they are close to the sides of the head with the palms flat, facing upward. Exhale and bend forward to touch the ground with the palms. As the hands touch the floor and the exhale is complete, pull in and up on the Root Lock. Inhale and straighten up, releasing the lock. Keep the arm and hand position intact as you bend and straighten. Continue very slowly with a deep breath for 1 to 2 minutes. Then increase the pace and continue more rapidly for 1 more minute.

TO BALANCE
THE HEAD AND HEART

This set helps to bring a balance between logic and feeling, between ideas and the "fire" to put them into action, between an overly intellectual mind and overly sensitive emotions. It aligns the head and heart, so you can be great and graceful, aware and loving.

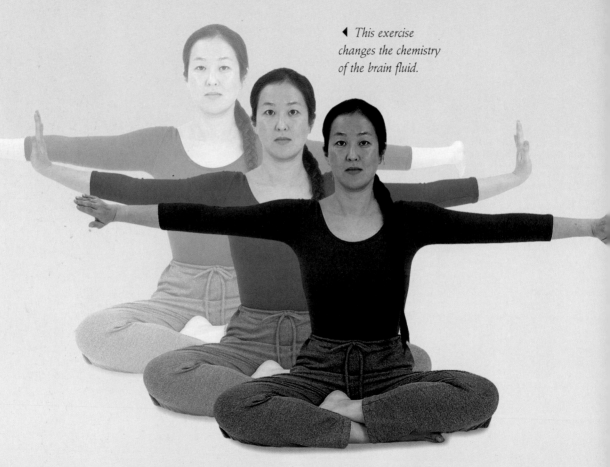

◀ *This exercise changes the chemistry of the brain fluid.*

1 Arm Twists Sit in Easy Pose, arms straight out to the sides from the shoulders with the wrists bent perpendicular to the arms, as though you were pressing the palms flat against two walls. There will be pressure on the wrists as you keep them pulled back in this position throughout the exercise. The beginning position is with the fingers facing straight up. This is the inhale position. Now exhale, and rotate the entire arm until the fingers face forward. Inhale and return to the beginning position. Then exhale again, and twist the arms until the fingers point backward. Then inhale in the beginning position. Continue, keeping all four movements distinct and separate. The elbows rotate. Move in a rhythm of 1 full cycle per 4 seconds. Continue for 3 to 7 minutes, then inhale, exhale, and relax. Massage the arms and shoulders for a few seconds.

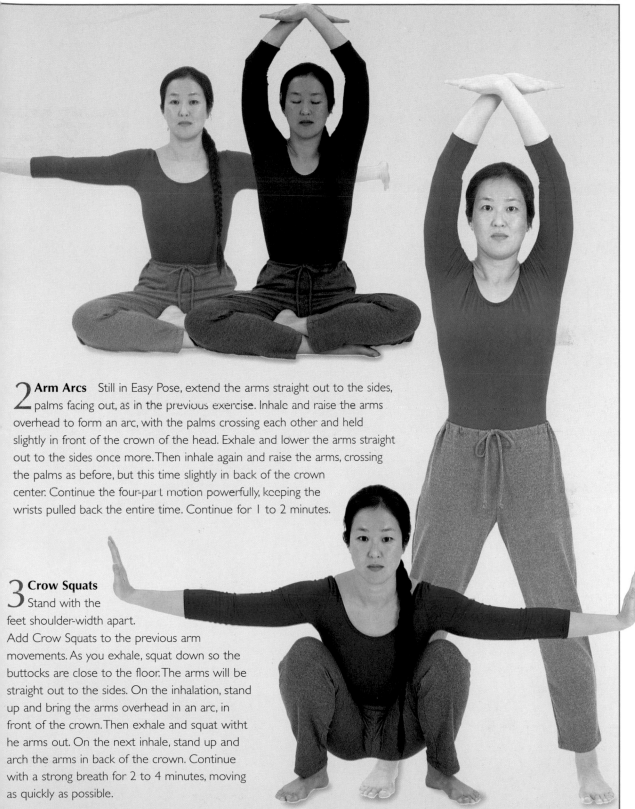

2 Arm Arcs   Still in Easy Pose, extend the arms straight out to the sides, palms facing out, as in the previous exercise. Inhale and raise the arms overhead to form an arc, with the palms crossing each other and held slightly in front of the crown of the head. Exhale and lower the arms straight out to the sides once more. Then inhale again and raise the arms, crossing the palms as before, but this time slightly in back of the crown center. Continue the four-part motion powerfully, keeping the wrists pulled back the entire time. Continue for 1 to 2 minutes.

3 Crow Squats
Stand with the feet shoulder-width apart. Add Crow Squats to the previous arm movements. As you exhale, squat down so the buttocks are close to the floor. The arms will be straight out to the sides. On the inhalation, stand up and bring the arms overhead in an arc, in front of the crown. Then exhale and squat witht he arms out. On the next inhale, stand up and arch the arms in back of the crown. Continue with a strong breath for 2 to 4 minutes, moving as quickly as possible.

FOR PHYSICAL AND MENTAL
VITALITY

When you want to work hard, this set delivers you to your own reserve of physical and mental vitality. It moves the kundalini energy from the lower chakras through to the higher centers. Mental projection and meditation are automatic afterward. The hard work brings deep relaxation and the experience that you have the latent power to cleanse and revitalize yourself.

1 Crisscross Lie down on your back and tip the pelvis forward, eliminating the arch in the spine. Using your abdominal muscles, lift your legs about 1 foot off the ground. Begin crisscrossing the legs, left over right then right over left, spreading the legs wide and keeping them straight the entire time. Inhale as they spread, exhale as they cross. Continue for 2 to 5 minutes. Then inhale, hold the legs up and apply the Root Lock. Exhale and relax the lock and the legs. Rest for 1 to 2 minutes, then repeat the cycle.

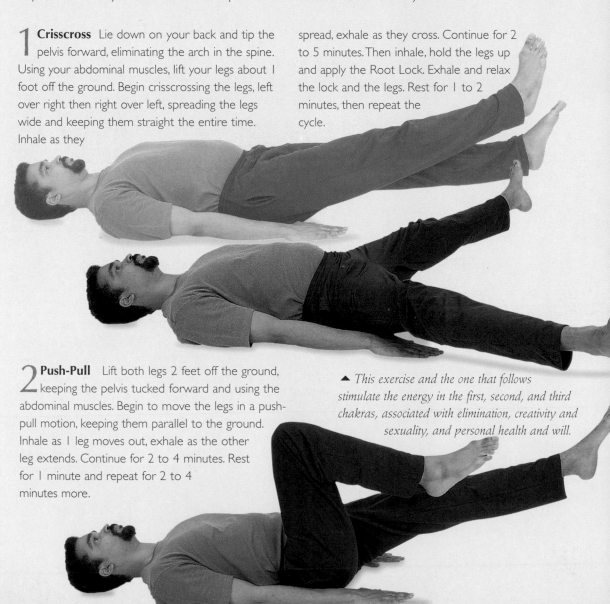

2 Push-Pull Lift both legs 2 feet off the ground, keeping the pelvis tucked forward and using the abdominal muscles. Begin to move the legs in a push-pull motion, keeping them parallel to the ground. Inhale as 1 leg moves out, exhale as the other leg extends. Continue for 2 to 4 minutes. Rest for 1 minute and repeat for 2 to 4 minutes more.

▲ *This exercise and the one that follows stimulate the energy in the first, second, and third chakras, associated with elimination, creativity and sexuality, and personal health and will.*

▶ *You are moving the kundalini energy from the first three chakras into the heart center with this exercise.*

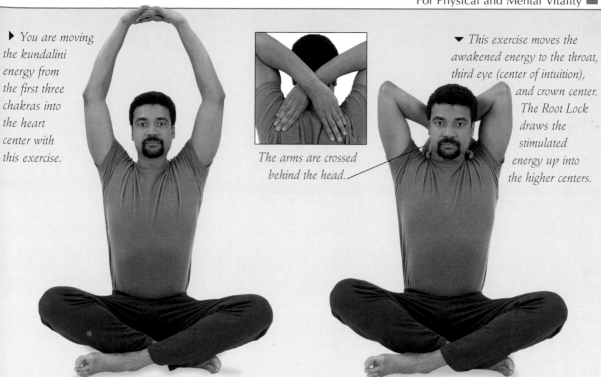

The arms are crossed behind the head.

▼ *This exercise moves the awakened energy to the throat, third eye (center of intuition), and crown center. The Root Lock draws the stimulated energy up into the higher centers.*

3 **Breathe and Stretch** Sitting in Easy Pose, interlock the fingers and stretch them straight overhead with the palms facing upward. Begin Breath of Fire for 2 to 5 minutes. Keep an upward stretch. Let all the worries of the day fall away. Feel that you are rising above the clouds and that your body is filled with the light energy of the breath.

4 **Light Energy** Still in Easy Pose, clasp opposite shoulders with the thumbs forward. The arms are crossed behind the head. Begin Breath of Fire for 2 to 5 minutes. Feel the light energy lift to your head and project your mind into an expansive peacefulness. Then inhale, exhale. Inhale again and hold the breath while feeling the energy circulating within you. Exhale and apply the Root Lock. Inhale, releasing the lock, and exhale. Repeat the sequence of inhaling, exhaling, and applying the Root Lock three more times. Then inhale, exhale, and relax.

5 **Relax** Relax completely on your back. Separate the mental body from the physical body, allowing the mind to be free to expand. Allow the physical body to rest peacefully for 10 minutes or so. Then bring yourself back by inhaling and exhaling deeply.

▼ *Be sure to finish with the wake-up exercises (page 183) to bring yourself back in a gentle, systematic way.*

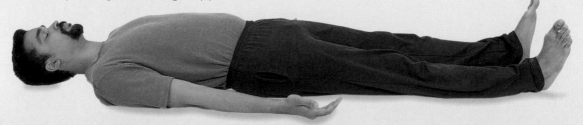

STRENGTHENING THE AURA

Your aura is the electromagnetic energy field that surrounds you. When the aura is weak a person feels readily swayed by others, overwhelmed by outside influences, and easily emotional. A strong aura gives you the power of protection (from outside influences and disease), and projection (clarity of intention). You feel stable and secure in your self. This allows you to shine and be openhearted.

This is a simple yet powerful kriya for keeping disease away, eliminating digestive problems, and developing a strong aura. The times can be gradually built to 7½ minutes for each side in the first exercise, and 15 minutes each for the last two exercises. This creates a tremendous, healing sweat.

◀ *This exercise moves energy into the upper body and upper chakras from the navel to the heart, the throat, and the third eye.*

1 **Yogic Push-Ups** Stand up. Bend forward, placing the hands on the ground shoulder-width apart. The body forms a triangle. Raise the right leg up with the knee straight. The body forms a continuous angle from the buttocks to the extended leg. Exhale and bend the elbows, bringing the head close to the ground. Inhale and raise the body up to the original position. Continue the push-ups, bending only the elbows, for 1½ minutes. Stand up and take a few deep breaths. Repeat the exercise, raising the left leg, for the same amount of time.

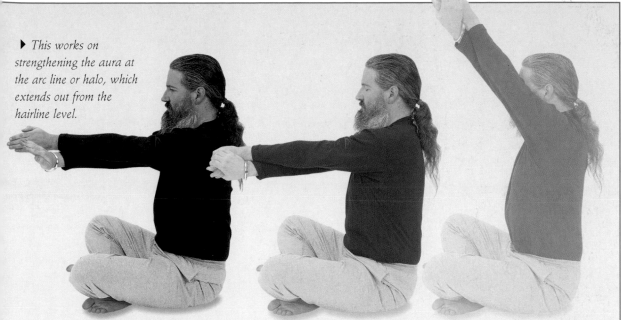

▶ *This works on strengthening the aura at the arc line or halo, which extends out from the hairline level.*

2 **Arm Raises** Sit in Easy Pose. Extend the left hand forward as if shaking hands. Bring the right hand underneath the left, and grasp the back of the left hand with the right. Lock the hands together. Both palms facing to the right. Inhale and raise the arms to a 60° angle above the horizontal. Exhale and return the arms to chest level. Continue this strong, chopping motion with a deep and powerful breath for 2 to 3 minutes, keeping the elbows straight. Then inhale, stretching the arms up. Exhale and relax.

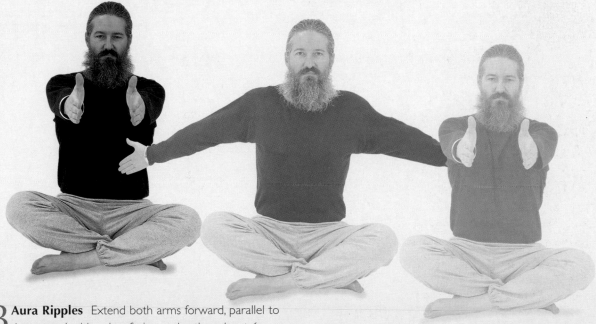

3 **Aura Ripples** Extend both arms forward, parallel to the ground with palms facing each other about 6 inches apart. As you inhale, open the arms, stretching them back and toward each other. They drop slightly as they open. Exhale and bring them forward to the original position. Use a deep, rhythmic breath and visualize your arms creating energy ripples that extend your aura further and further. Continue for 2 to 3 minutes.

FOR A HEALTHY
MENTAL BALANCE

This powerful set activates and balances the body's energy. It begins with backward bending poses to energize and open the upper back and chest. The next few excercises circulate the energy to the brain, concluding with a powerful meditation to balance the mind. Be sure to rest after this kriya.

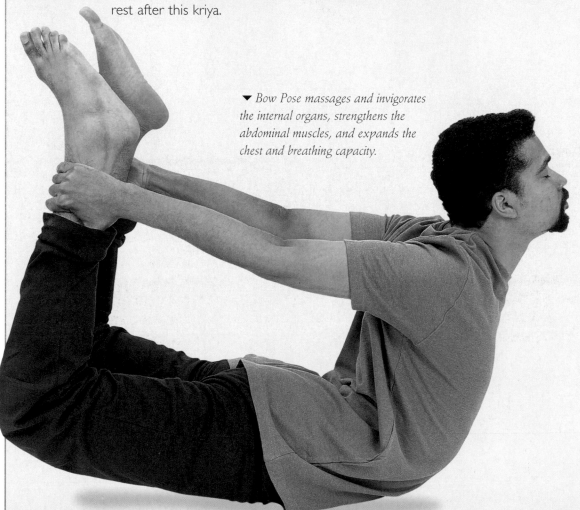

▼ *Bow Pose massages and invigorates the internal organs, strengthens the abdominal muscles, and expands the chest and breathing capacity.*

1 **Bow Pose with Lion Breath**   Lying on your stomach, reach back and hold onto the ankles. Arch your body up as you inhale, lifting the head, chest, and thighs off the floor. Stretch the head back to lift the chest further. Create a tension between the straight arms and the legs to stretch higher. Breathe deeply for 1 to 2 minutes. Then, with the tongue pulled out as far as possible, breathe heavily through your mouth. This breath is called the Breath of the Lion. Continue for 1 to 1½ minutes more. Then inhale, exhale, and relax down.

▼ *Besides bringing great flexibility to the spine, Camel Pose adjusts the navel point and relieves the stomach from the effects of overeating. Regular practice gives control over hunger and thirst.*

▼ *Both Bow and Camel Poses stretch the thigh muscle, which controls the calcium-magnesium balance in the body. This balance is necessary for both physical and mental well-being.*

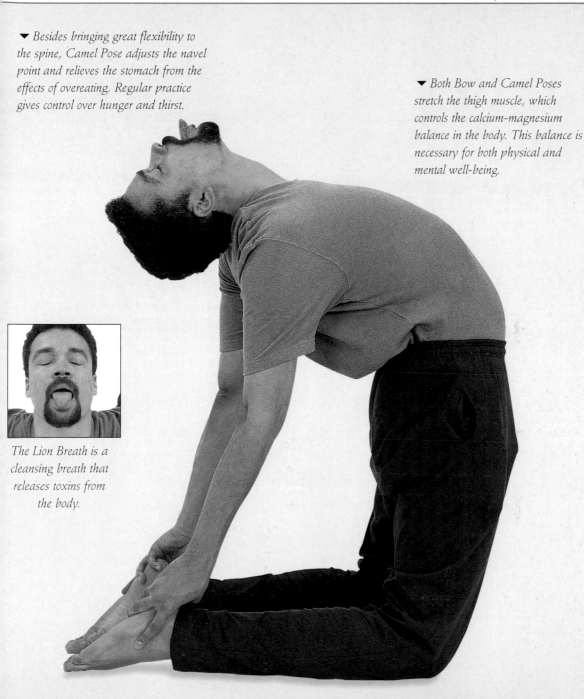

The Lion Breath is a cleansing breath that releases toxins from the body.

2 **Camel Pose** Sit on the heels in Rock Pose. Reach back and take hold of the heels. Using the abdominal muscles, arch the body up, keeping the arms straight. The chest is lifted upward, and the head is dropped back. Press the hips forward to steady the pose. Once again, stretch out the tongue as far as possible and begin Lion Breath. Continue for 1 to 2 minutes.

3 **Frog Pose** Stand up with the heels close together and the feet spread outward. Squat down with the buttocks close to the heels, and the hands on the ground in front of you. The arms are between the knees, which are open. Sit up straight. Ideally the heels remain slightly off the floor as you inhale and straighten the legs, bringing the head down and close to the knees. Exhale and squat down into the original position. Continue at your own pace for a count of 26 to 108 frogs (up-and-down counts as 1). Inhale, then exhale and relax sitting down. Stretch the legs out in front of you and shake them for a few seconds. Relax.

▼ *Frog Pose stimulates the energy of the first three chakras, associated with elimination, creativity and sexuality, and personal health and will. It then moves and circulates the energy to the heart and higher centers.*

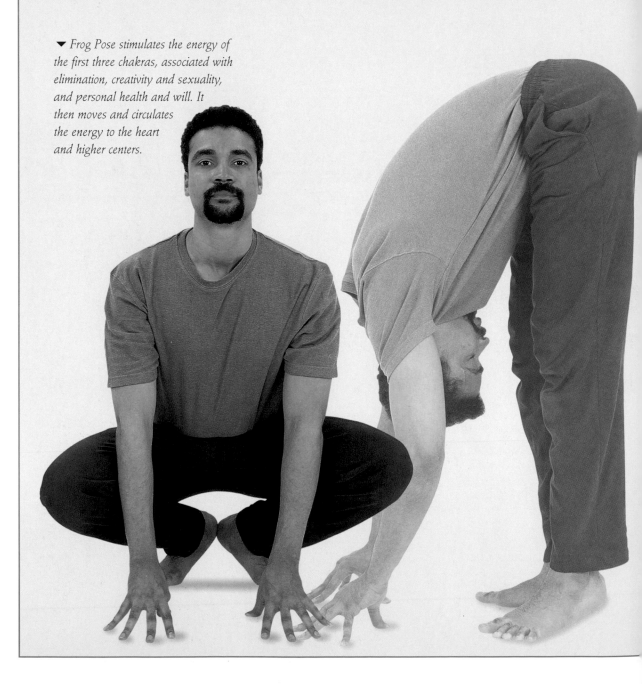

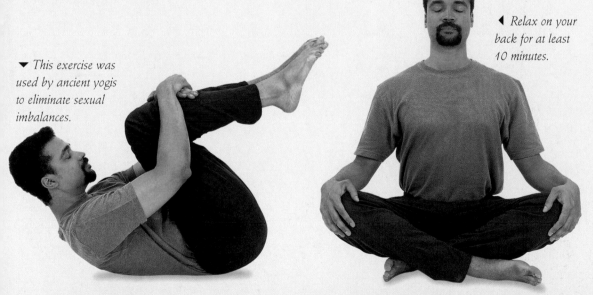

To help sit in Celibate Pose, use a small but firm pillow under the buttocks. This will ease some of the pressure on the hips and knees.

4 Celibate Pose From a position of sitting on your heels, move your heels out to the sides so that your buttocks are resting on the floor. Spread your knees as far apart as possible. Clasp your hands behind your back with the fingers interlaced. From this position lower your torso forward to the floor and rise back up, moving your shoulders from side to side, weaving like a snake. Continue for 1 to 3 minutes.

◀ *Relax on your back for at least 10 minutes.*

▼ *This exercise was used by ancient yogis to eliminate sexual imbalances.*

5 Tuck and Bounce Lie on your back. Bring the knees to the chest and lock the arms around the shins. While holding in this position, bounce your body up and down on the floor. Continue for 2 to 7 minutes.

6 Power Breath Sit in Easy Pose with the spine straight, the neck in line with the spine, and the chin slightly tucked in. Rest the hands on the knees. Inhale and powerfully exhale so that the sound of the breath leaving the nostrils sounds like the mantra *Har* (The Infinite One). Press the navel toward the spine on the exhalation so that you feel the force all the way from the navel to the nostrils. The rib cage lifts with the power of the breath. Continue for 2 to 5 minutes.

LET THE LIVER LIVE

The liver performs the great service of removing toxins from the bloodstream, but if the liver becomes overtaxed the whole body will suffer. This yoga set focuses on preventative care of the liver.

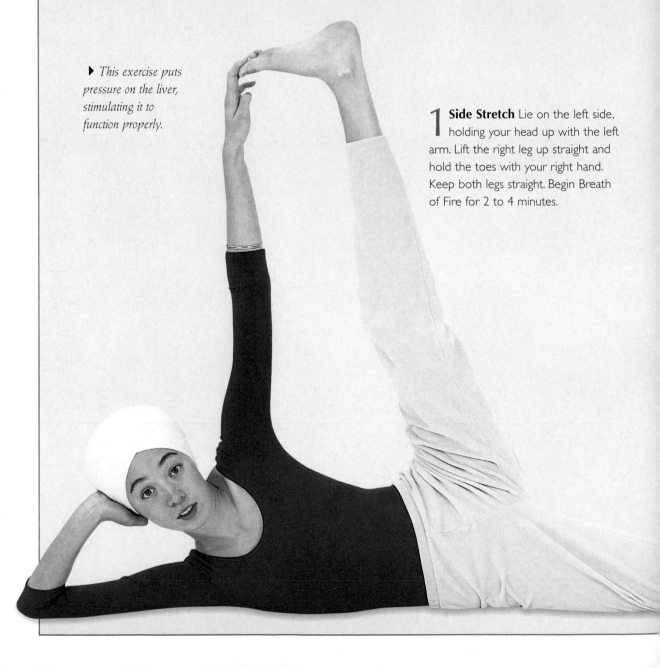

▶ *This exercise puts pressure on the liver, stimulating it to function properly.*

1 Side Stretch Lie on the left side, holding your head up with the left arm. Lift the right leg up straight and hold the toes with your right hand. Keep both legs straight. Begin Breath of Fire for 2 to 4 minutes.

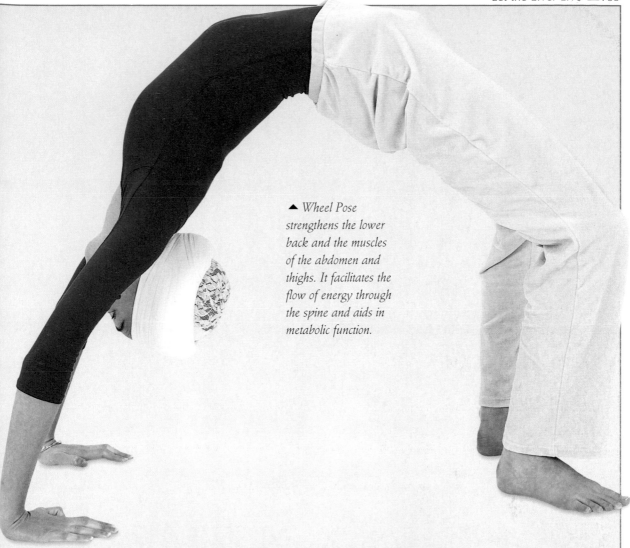

▲ *Wheel Pose strengthens the lower back and the muscles of the abdomen and thighs. It facilitates the flow of energy through the spine and aids in metabolic function.*

2 **Wheel Pose** Lie on the back. Bend the legs with the soles of the feet pressed against the floor close to the buttocks. Bending the elbows, place the palms of the hands on the floor above the shoulders, with the fingers pointing back toward the shoulders. Keeping the feet and knees parallel, begin to carefully lift the body off the floor by pushing against the floor with the hands and feet. Lead with the hips, followed by the chest. The neck will arch back as you straighten the elbows. The body will form one continuous arch from the heels to the hands. Breathe in and out through the nose, then in and out through the mouth. Continue alternating between nose and mouth breathing for 1 to 4 minutes. (See page 85 for an alternative to Wheel Pose.)

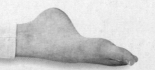

3 **Side Stretch** Repeat the first exercise of the kriya, Side Stretch, for 1 to 2 minutes.

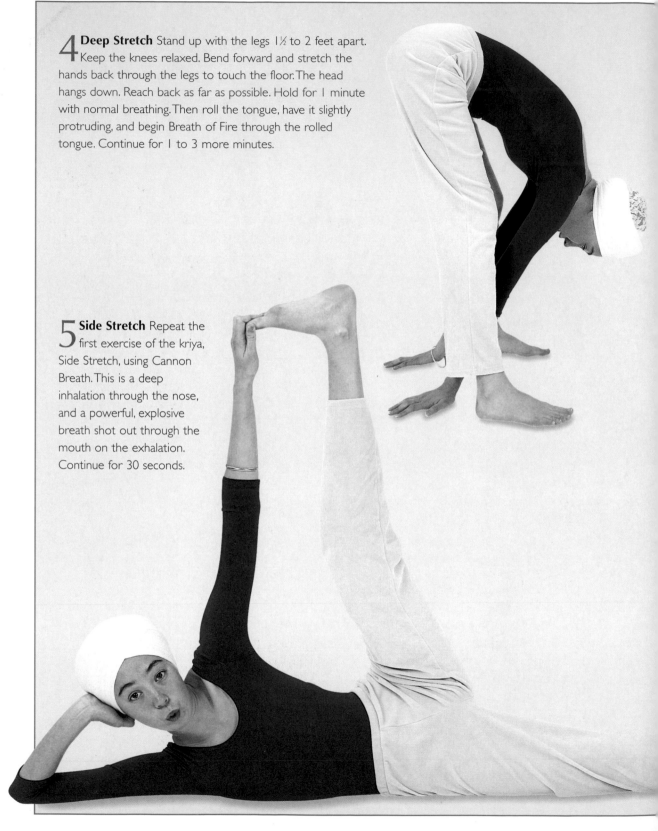

4 **Deep Stretch** Stand up with the legs 1½ to 2 feet apart. Keep the knees relaxed. Bend forward and stretch the hands back through the legs to touch the floor. The head hangs down. Reach back as far as possible. Hold for 1 minute with normal breathing. Then roll the tongue, have it slightly protruding, and begin Breath of Fire through the rolled tongue. Continue for 1 to 3 more minutes.

5 **Side Stretch** Repeat the first exercise of the kriya, Side Stretch, using Cannon Breath. This is a deep inhalation through the nose, and a powerful, explosive breath shot out through the mouth on the exhalation. Continue for 30 seconds.

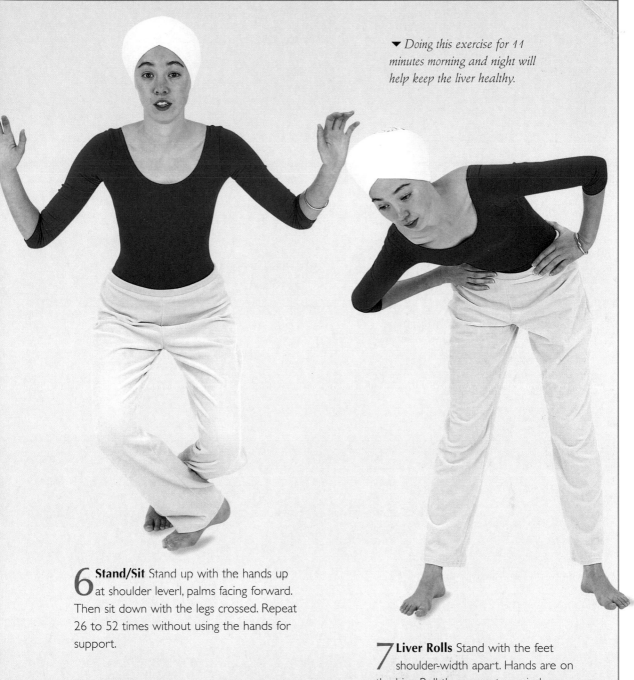

▼ *Doing this exercise for 11 minutes morning and night will help keep the liver healthy.*

6 **Stand/Sit** Stand up with the hands up at shoulder leverl, palms facing forward. Then sit down with the legs crossed. Repeat 26 to 52 times without using the hands for support.

7 **Liver Rolls** Stand with the feet shoulder-width apart. Hands are on the hips. Roll the upper torso in large circles. Inhale as you come around one side, exhale around the other. After 1 minute, reverse the direction, and continue for 1 more minute.

TO RELIEVE
INNER ANGER

Inner anger blocks your relationships with others because it blocks your relationship with yourself. This powerful set works to effectively release and transform inner anger.

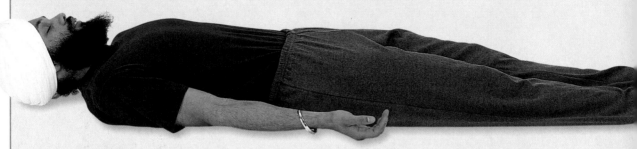

1 Sleep Pose Lie down on your back in a relaxed posture with your arms at your side, palms up, and your legs slightly apart. Close the eyes and pretend to snore. Continue for 1½ minutes.

▼ *This exercise balances anger. It applies pressure to the navel to balance the entire system.*

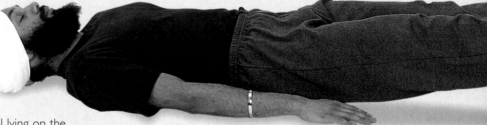

2 Leg Hold #1 Still lying on the back, keep your legs straight and raise both legs 6 inches above the ground and hold. Breathe normally for to 2 minutes.

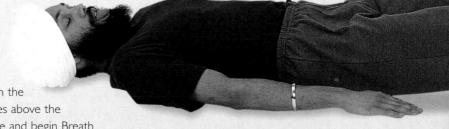

3 Leg Hold #2 Still lying on the back with the legs 6 inches above the ground, stretch out the tongue and begin Breath of Fire through the mouth for 1½ minutes.

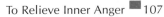

4 Beat the Ground Still lying on the back, lift the legs perpendicular to the floor, resting the arms on the ground by the sides, palms down. Begin to beat the ground with all the anger you can achieve. Beat hard and fast, using the entire length of the arms. Continue for 2½ minutes.

5 Knees to Chest Bring the knees to the chest and wrap the arms around them. Stretch the tongue out. Inhale through the open mouth, exhale through the nose. Continue for 1 to 2 minutes.

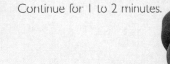

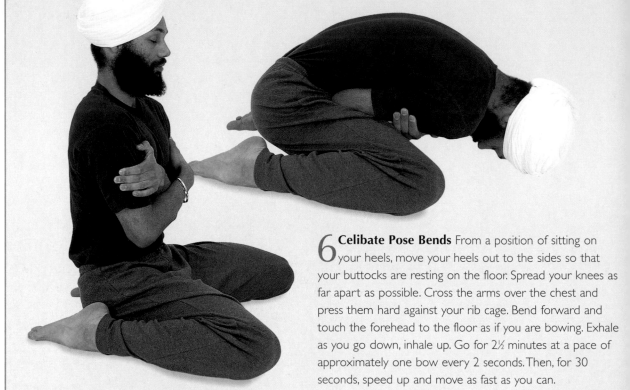

6 Celibate Pose Bends From a position of sitting on your heels, move your heels out to the sides so that your buttocks are resting on the floor. Spread your knees as far apart as possible. Cross the arms over the chest and press them hard against your rib cage. Bend forward and touch the forehead to the floor as if you are bowing. Exhale as you go down, inhale up. Go for 2½ minutes at a pace of approximately one bow every 2 seconds. Then, for 30 seconds, speed up and move as fast as you can.

Sat Kriya

Stretch the arms up with the elbows hugging the sides of the head. Interlock all the fingers except the index fingers of each hand, which are pointing straight up. Begin to say the sound *sat* as you pull the navel up and in toward the spine. As you say *nam*, relax the belly area. Chant emphatically in a constant rhythm about 8 times per 10 seconds. Then, inhale and squeeze the muscles tightly from the buttocks all the way up the back, past the shoulders. Mentally allow the energy to flow through the head and out the top of the skull. Exhale and relax.

This exercise circulates the kundalini energy and integrates the energy released from the lower three chakras into the entire system, so that the total effects of these exercises are stable and long lasting.

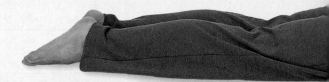

9 Cobra Pose Lie on the stomach with the palms flat on the floor under the shoulders. The heels are together, and the tops of the feet are on the floor. Inhale into Cobra Pose, stretching the spine, vertebra by vertebra, from the neck to the base of the spine as far as possible. The arms may be slightly bent at the elbow to ensure that the shoulders are not tensed. Make sure to stretch the head out of the neck,

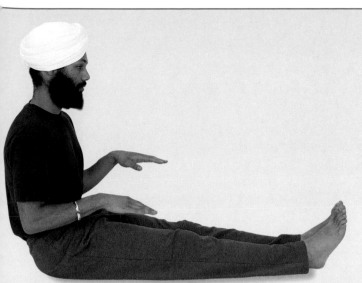

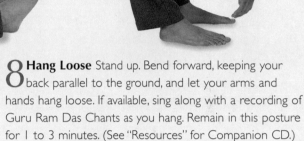

7 **Self-Massage** Sit with the legs straight out in front of you. Begin to beat all parts of your body with open palms. Move quickly for 2 minutes.

8 **Hang Loose** Stand up. Bend forward, keeping your back parallel to the ground, and let your arms and hands hang loose. If available, sing along with a recording of Guru Ram Das Chants as you hang. Remain in this posture for 1 to 3 minutes. (See "Resources" for Companion CD.)

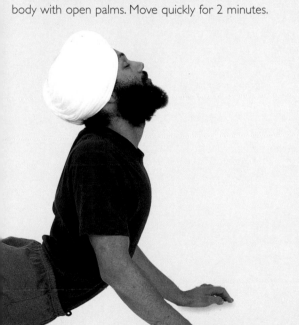

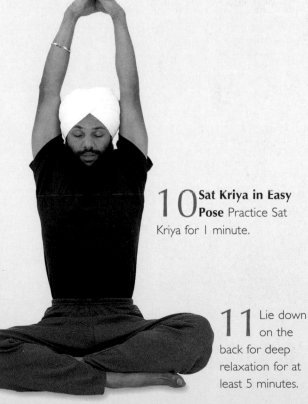

10 **Sat Kriya in Easy Pose** Practice Sat Kriya for 1 minute.

and relax the shoulders downward. Exhale. Continue to sing with the Guru Ram Das Chant, if possible, while stretching into Cobra for 1 minute. Then, still in Cobra and singing, begin to circle the head around on the neck both ways for a total of 30 seconds. Still in Cobra Pose, begin kicking the ground with alternate feet. Continue for 30 seconds.

11 Lie down on the back for deep relaxation for at least 5 minutes.

FOR A NEW
ENERGY BALANCE

As human beings, we have certain animal instincts, but we also have the ability to direct, shape, and give meaning to the expression of these instincts. Many of the strongest instincts find expression through the "lower triangle" of energy centers, or chakras. These are the first, second, and third chakras, which correspond in the body as the rectal, sexual, and navel centers.

To change learned patterns that no longer serve us, this yoga set, or kriya, first activates the lower triangle. Next the activated energy is raised to the higher centers of the heart, throat, third-eye point or intuitive center, and crown. Once this is achieved, a new energy balance is attained which allows you to balance all of your chakras, and elevate yourself. Remember to bring your mind to focus on what you are doing and experiencing during each moment of this kriya.

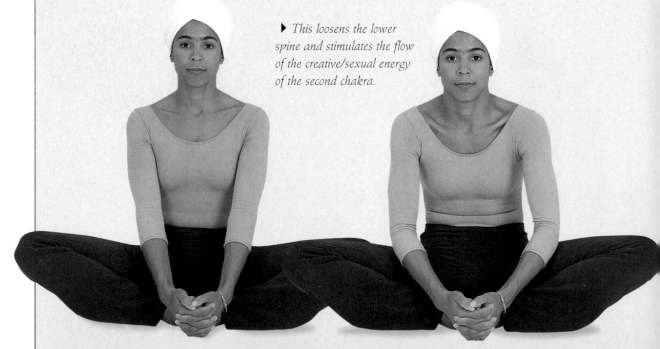

▶ *This loosens the lower spine and stimulates the flow of the creative/sexual energy of the second chakra.*

1 **Spine Flex** Sit with the soles of the feet pressed together. Hold the feet with both hands and draw them into the groin, keeping the knees as close to the floor as possible. Inhale and flex the spine forward, keeping the head straight and chest out. Exhale and curve the spine back, rounding the shoulders. Continue rhythmically, coordinating the movement with the breath for 1 to 3 minutes. Inhale and hold the breath briefly, exhale and relax.

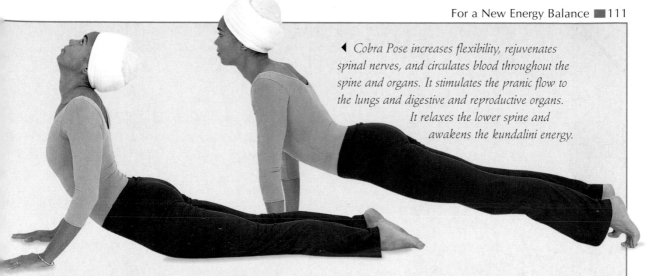

◀ *Cobra Pose increases flexibility, rejuvenates spinal nerves, and circulates blood throughout the spine and organs. It stimulates the pranic flow to the lungs and digestive and reproductive organs. It relaxes the lower spine and awakens the kundalini energy.*

2 **Cobra/Platform** Lie on the stomach with the palms flat under the shoulders. The tops of the feet are on the floor, heels together. Inhale into Cobra Pose, (see page 54). Exhale. On the next inhalation, position the feet so that the underside of the toes are pressing the floor, and raise the body up so that it forms a straight line from the head to the heels. The arms are straight. This is Back Platform. Exhale and lower the body back into Cobra Pose. Continue alternating between Cobra and Back Platform rhythmically with powerful breathing for 1 to 3 minutes. Then inhale into Cobra Pose, hold the breath briefly, and focus inwardly, pulling the Root Lock (see page 35). Exhale, relax, and come down. Turn the head to the side and rest for 30 seconds.

▶ *This exercise circulates the energy of the lower three chakras and opens up the circulation to the hips and intestines.*

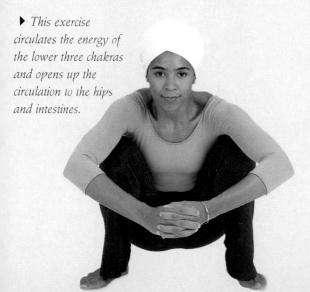

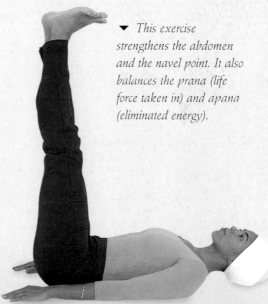

▼ *This exercise strengthens the abdomen and the navel point. It also balances the prana (life force taken in) and apana (eliminated energy).*

3 **Crow Pose** Stand with the feet shoulder-width apart. Crouch down so that the buttocks are as close to the floor as possible. The soles of the feet should be flat on the floor. Keep the spine straight. Wrap the arms around the knees with the hands in Venus Lock (see page 31). Begin Breath of Fire. Continue for 1 to 3 minutes. Inhale. Exhale and relax.

4 **Leg Raises** Lie on your back. Inhale and raise the legs to a 90° angle from the floor (straight up). Exhale and lower the legs. Continue with powerful deep breathing for 1 to 3 minutes.

5 **Extended Locust Pose** Lie on the stomach. Interlock the fingers in Venus Lock at the small of the back. Inhale, raising the head, arms, and legs as far as possible. Pull up with minimal bending. Begin Breath of Fire. Continue for 1 to 3 minutes. Inhale, exhale, and relax.

▼ *This exercise strengthens the lower back, allows the energy to flow to the mid-spine, and opens the nerve channels in the area of the solar plexus.*

6 **Relax and Rock** Relax on the back for 1 to 3 minutes with the arms at the sides and the palms facing up. Then pull the knees to the chest and wrap the arms around them. Press the head forward, bringing the nose between the knees. Rock back and forth on the spine from the base to the top for 1 minute.

▼ *These exercises relax the spine and distribute the energy from the previous exercises.*

7 **Shoulder Stand into Plow Pose** Lie on the back. Raise the legs to a 90° angle. Then, using the arms for support, begin to push the body gently up by walking the hands up the back toward the shoulders. As you relax in this pose stretch up higher on the shoulders, adjusting the supporting hand position. Begin Breath of Fire for 1 to 3 minutes. Now, continuing Breath of Fire, slowly lower the legs back behind you in Plow Pose. Continue to support the body with the hands. If you can reach the floor, be on the balls of the feet with the heels stretched away from you. A wall can be used for support if the feet do not reach the floor. Rest the arms down on the floor with the palms facing downward and flat. Continue Breath of Fire for 1 to 2 minutes. Inhale deeply. Exhale and relax the breath. Slowly come out of the posture by either supporting yourself with the hands on the floor or on your back. Take a full 30 seconds to come out of the pose, exhaling slowly and massaging each vertebra against the floor. Relax on your back for a minute.

◄ *These exercises open the upper spine and related nerve passages to the flow of kundalini energy. They also strengthen and balance the thyroid and parathyroid glands.*

8 Sat Kriya Sit between the heels in Celibate Pose, or, if you prefer, sit on the heels. Stretch the arms straight overhead so that the elbows hug the ears. Interlock all the fingers except the index fingers, which are placed together and pointing straight up. Begin to say the sound *Sat* as you pull the navel up and in toward the spine. As you say *Nam*, relax the belly area. Chant emphatically in a constant rhythm, about 8 times per 10 seconds. Continue for 3 to 5 minutes. Then inhale and squeeze the muscles tightly from the buttocks all the way up the back, past the shoulders. Mentally allow the energy to flow through the head and out the top of the skull. Exhale and relax.

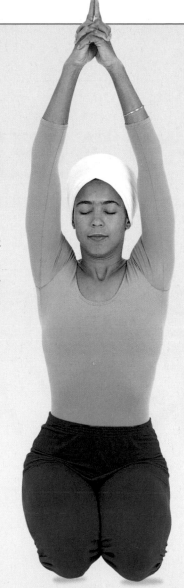

◀ *This exercise circulates the kundalini energy and integrates the energy released from the lower three chakras into the entire system, so that the total effects of these exercises are stable and long lasting.*

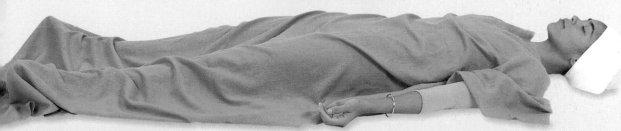

▲ *Deep relaxation after a yoga set is essential. It allows you to enjoy and consciously integrate the internal changes brought about by the kriya. If you have a light shawl, cover yourself so the body maintains a constant temperature. Allow your physical body to deeply relax with long, light breathing, and sense the extension of the self through your energy field, or aura.*

9 Relaxation Deeply relax on the back for 5 to 10 minutes.

CHAPTER 5

INTERMEDIATE
KRIYAS

"Keep up and you'll be kept up."
–Yogi Bhajan

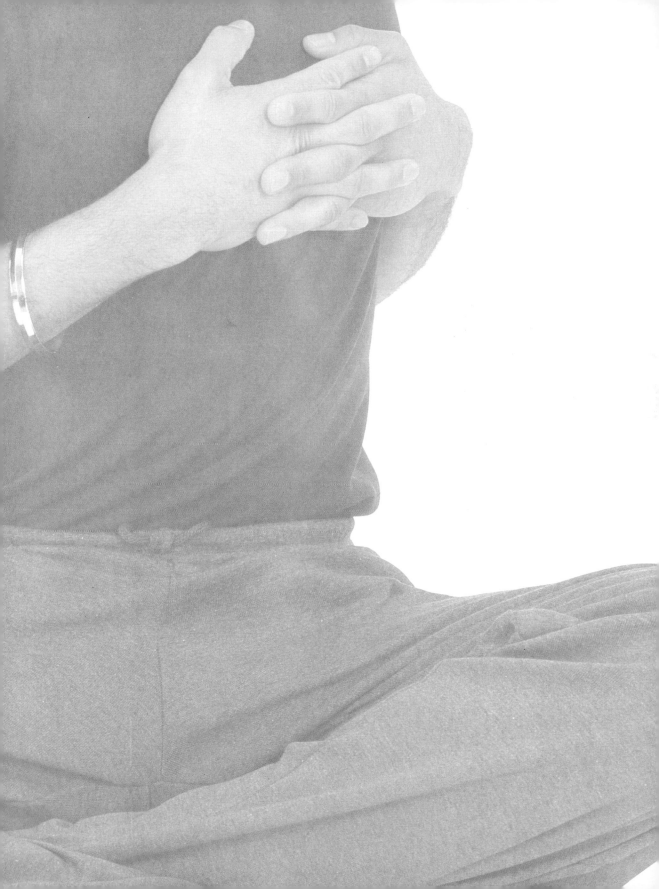

A DEFINITION OF
INTERMEDIATE KRIYAS

This section of kriyas has been given by Yogi Bhajan in the more recent past. They are on an intermediate level in a number of ways: the physical stamina required; the longer length of times given; the types of breathing patterns or combinations of breath and mantra; and the subtlety of their effects. They were designed to match the vibratory energy of the age our world is moving into, although all Kundalini Yoga is of a timeless nature.

Begin practicing with the minimum times given. Refer to the "Resources" section for helpful aids, such as meditation music and further tools of study of Kundalini Yoga.

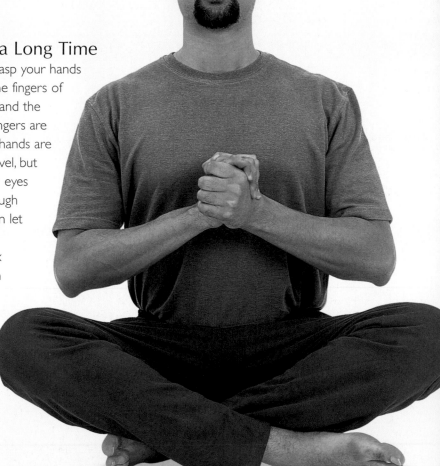

To Live Young for a Long Time

Sit with a straight spine. Clasp your hands together and lock them. The fingers of the right hand are on top, and the thumbs are crossed. The fingers are not interlaced. The locked hands are held at the heart-center level, but not touching the body. The eyes are closed. Breathe in through the mouth in 3 strokes, then let it out through the nose in 1 breath. Squeeze and relax your locked hands on each stroke of the inhalation. Perform 3 squeezes for 1 complete breath. Do not squeeze on the exhale. Press the two hands very consciously. Continue for 15 minutes.

To complete the meditation, inhale, make your hand grip very tight, and squeeze your entire body. Bring the energy to a central balance system. Hold the breath for 20 seconds, then breathe out with a Cannon Breath through the mouth. Inhale again. Bring your shoulders, arms, feet, spine, your whole self, into one solid iron-like state. Hold for 20 seconds, then breathe out with Cannon Breath. Inhale once more. Do nothing this time, just suspend the breath with your will for 20 seconds. Then exhale and relax.

We are responsible for our health and energy. Breath is the source of life. How much we stimulate [it], that is the deciding factor.

–Yogi Bhajan

▶ *This meditation is a pranayam, which means that it uses a powerful yogic breathing technique. Apply the mind very consciously as you coordinate the hand movement and breath. It works on the total health of the being, giving the vitality to live young for a long time.*

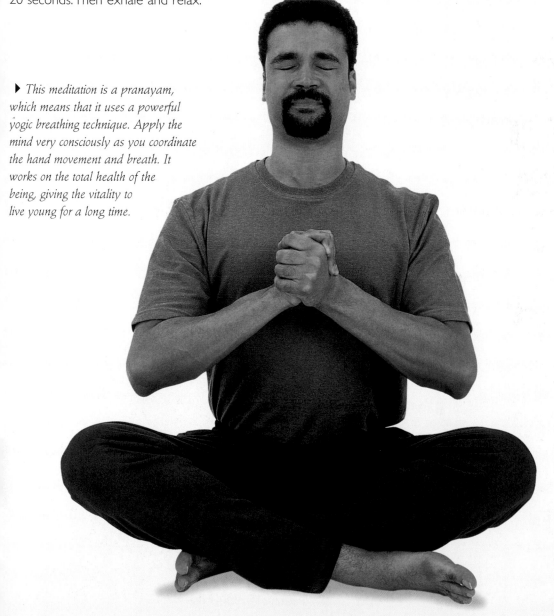

SEVEN STEPS TO HEALTH

Here is a sample of a physical-training class given by Yogi Bhajan at the Khalsa Women's Training Camp in New Mexico in the summer of 1994. KWTC is a camp that began in 1976 to give women a place to relax, rejuvenate, and experience their excellence. Khalsa is the Gurmukhi name for the pure spirit that is every human's birthright.

This yoga set is a vigorous workout that will revitalize you in a short time. Eventually, you can extend the meditation time to a maximum of 31 minutes. Start with 11 minutes, and as your practice grows, increase the time gradually.

▶ *This movement rejuvenates the brain, spine, and nervous system.*

1 Lower Spine Stretch Stand with the hands on the hips, legs spread slightly. Keep the knees relaxed. Stretch the spine forward. Focus on stretching out the lower spine. Press the hips and buttocks away from you as you elongate and stretch the spine, which will be almost parallel to the ground. Breathe normally. Continue for 2 minutes.

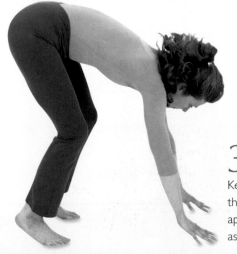

2 Hammer Circle Return to a standing position. Bend over and let the arms hang loosely in front of you. Begin to straighten the body slightly, swinging the torso and arms to the right. Straighten fully, and circle your arms straight up over your head, then bend and swing down to the left and back to the center starting position. Stop when you return to the front and then circle 1 time to the left. Again, stop when circle is complete. Continue alternating directions. Breathe rhythmically, inhaling as you begin your circle, exhaling as you come back around to the front. Continue for 2 minutes.

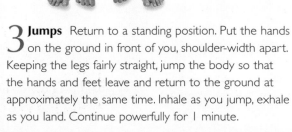

3 Jumps Return to a standing position. Put the hands on the ground in front of you, shoulder-width apart. Keeping the legs fairly straight, jump the body so that the hands and feet leave and return to the ground at approximately the same time. Inhale as you jump, exhale as you land. Continue powerfully for 1 minute.

4 **Swaying Tree** Stand with legs shoulder-width apart, knees slightly bent. Raise the arms up with palms facing forward, hands open for balance. Lean forward at an approximately 30° angle, then lean backward at a 30° angle (or less). Sway like a tree in the breeze, leaning equally forward and backward. The movement should involve the lower body as well – try as best you can to sway from the legs through the torso. Continue for 1 minute.

5 **Leap Run** Begin to run in a large circle. With every step, leap high. Use your arms to add power to your leap. Continue for 4 minutes.

6 **Pradhan Kriya** Sit in Easy Pose and normalize your breath by breathing deeply. Then bring your arms up so that the bent elbows are close to the ribs and the hands are approximately at neck level. The palms of the hands are open and facing forward. Stretch out the chest and straighten the spine. With the eyes closed, imagine you are looking at the tip of the nose. Chant either *Har* (the Infinite One) or *Wahe Guru* (the ecstatic expression of union with infinity.

Begin with 7 minutes in this pose, gradually increasing over time to a maximum of 31 minutes.

Alternatives

Note: The following two mudras can be used in place of Pradhan Kriya in this same meditation:

• Gian Kriya •

Arms are in the same position as in Pradhan Kriya, but make fists of the hands with only the index fingers stretched up, pointing toward the sky.

• Dyan Kriya •

The arms are bent so that the hands are at neck level, with the palms facing down. For women, the left arm is over the right with 3 to 4 inches of space between them. The hand position is reversed for men. Balance the arms equally. The eyes look at the tip of the nose in a soft gaze.

7 **Stretching Set** The following is all one exercise, even though it has many parts. Each part is brief. Times given are approximate.

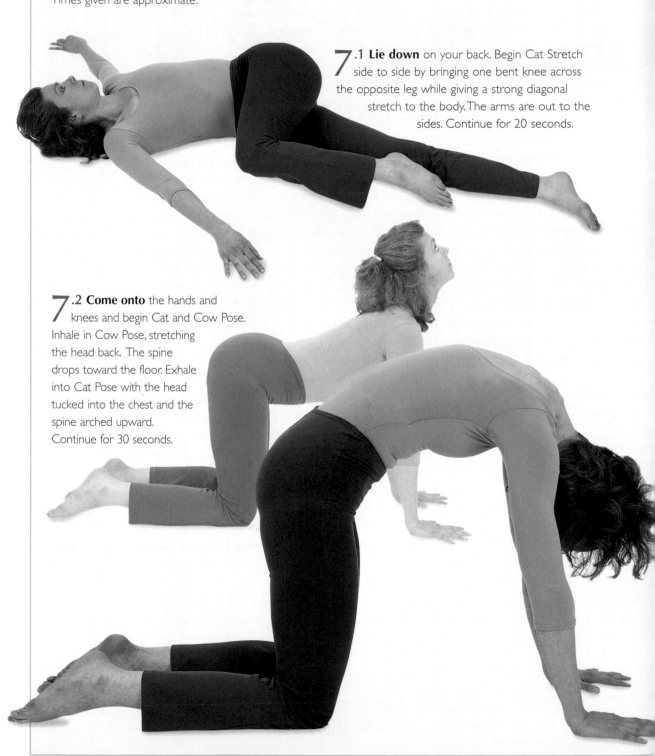

7.1 **Lie down** on your back. Begin Cat Stretch side to side by bringing one bent knee across the opposite leg while giving a strong diagonal stretch to the body. The arms are out to the sides. Continue for 20 seconds.

7.2 **Come onto** the hands and knees and begin Cat and Cow Pose. Inhale in Cow Pose, stretching the head back. The spine drops toward the floor. Exhale into Cat Pose with the head tucked into the chest and the spine arched upward. Continue for 30 seconds.

7.3 Lie down on the stomach. Place the hands on the ground overhead. Take a 1-minute nap.

7.4 Do a Bundle Twist Roll over onto your back by tightening the entire body and rocking back and forth until you flip over. Then stand up.

7.5 Bend forward and touch the ground.

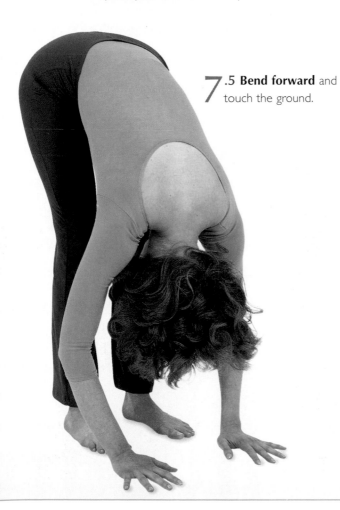

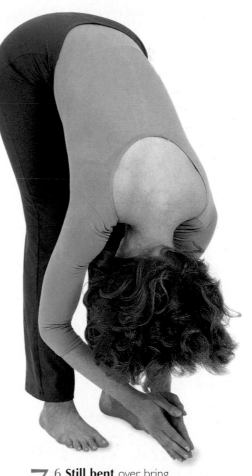

7.6 Still bent over, bring the palms together in Prayer Pose. Stabilize yourself. Make a 1-second prayer. Then stand up.

YOUR TEN BODIES

The human psyche is composed of ten separate but interrelated bodies. With the exception of one body, the physical, these bodies are made of light energy. Each of your ten bodies has a gift it gives when activated. Conversely, each brings specific challenges when in a weakened state. Through understanding your ten bodies, and using yoga and meditation to strengthen them, they become tools to help you reach your highest potential.

There is an ancient yogic science called Tantric or Akara Numerology, which is a system for understanding how our ten bodies work in our lives. Through simple calculations based on our individual birthdays, inherent strengths and challenges are revealed. Through Kundalini Yoga and meditation, these challenges can be changed into strengths. For example, if a person born in the month of September (ninth month) wanted to work on the challenge of that number's position, he or she could practice the yoga set called *Wahe Guru Kriya*, which strengthens the Subtle (ninth) body. (For more information, see Numerology entries in the "Resources" section.)

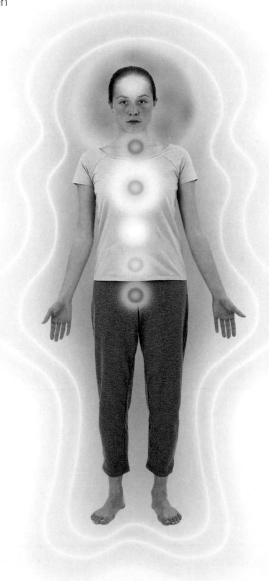

You are a human being: *hu* means "halo, light"; *man* means "mind, mental"; *being* means "now." If you understand that you are ten bodies, and you are aware of those ten bodies, and you keep them in balance, the whole universe will be in balance with you.

–Yogi Bhajan

THE TEN BODIES AND HOW THEY FUNCTION

First Body, the Soul: Relates to the first chakra, the root chakra. It is the Infinite Light that lives within you, and is your very best friend.
Challenge: To balance the head and heart.

Second Body, the Mental Negative: Relates to the second chakra. The Negative Mind protects you by revealing the danger or loss in any situation. It gives you the gifts of containment and discernment.
Challenge: Tendency to see things in a negative light.

Third Body, the Mental Positive: Relates to the navel center. The Positive Mind inspires you by telling you what the possible gain is in any situation.
Challenge: Tendency toward idealism, or can succumb to the negative mind.

Fourth Body, the Mental Neutral: Relates to the heart center. The Neutral Mind listens to both the Negative and Positive Minds, and then leads you to the best decision.
Challenge: Tendency toward indecision, or difficulty perceiving the larger picture.

Fifth Body, the Physical: Relates to the throat chakra. Your physical body is where the other light bodies play out their parts. It is the "teacher," one who can take the abstract and make it concrete and practical.
Challenge: When the fifth body is weak, the inner and outer realities will tend to be out of balance.

Sixth Body, the Arc Line: A ribbon of energy that arcs from earlobe to earlobe (a "halo"). It gives the ability to focus, to meditate, and to manifest projected thoughts and desires.
Challenge: Weakness shows up in difficulties in meditating, focusing, and using the intuition.

Seventh Body, the Aura: The sphere of electromagnetic energy that surrounds the physical body and can extend up to 9 feet in every direction. When the aura is strong, no disease, including negativity from others, can penetrate, and that person is completely confident and secure.
Challenge: Tendency to feel easily overwhelmed by outside influence, or to be an "energy drain" on others.

Eighth Body, the Pranic: Controls the breath and takes in prana, the life-force energy of the universe. When the Pranic Body is working, you are fearless and fully alive. Your pranic energy heals others.
Challenge: Tendency to be fearful, exhibit defensive behavior when weak, or to feel sluggish and fatigued.

Ninth Body, the Subtle: Carries the soul when it leaves the body. When the Subtle Body is strong, you see beyond the obvious and nothing in life is a mystery. It gives great finesse and a powerful calmness.
Challenge: When the Subtle Body is weak, a person may be naive and easily fooled, and unintentionally crude or unrefined in speech and behavior.

Tenth Body, the Radiant: A glorious, radiant sphere of light that gives you spiritual royalty and grace. You exert a magnetic presence that can heal others even at a distance.
Challenge: A tendency toward fear of conflict and ineffectiveness in life.

The Command Center: The center from which you direct the play of the ten bodies. From here, you master all ten bodies and can use them as needed to excel in your own life, and to help uplift others.

AWAKENING TO
YOUR TEN BODIES

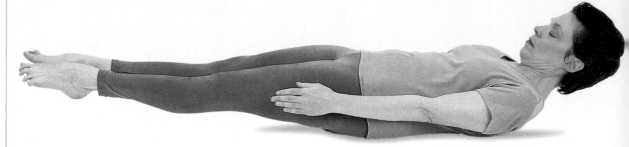

1 Stretch Pose Lie down on your back. Tip the pelvis forward, then bring the feet together and raise them 6 inches from the ground, keeping the legs straight. Raise your head 6 inches and fix your eyes on the toes, which point away from you. Arms are held straight at your sides, palms facing the thighs but not touching. Hold this position for 2 to 3 minutes while performing Breath of Fire. Relax for a few seconds.

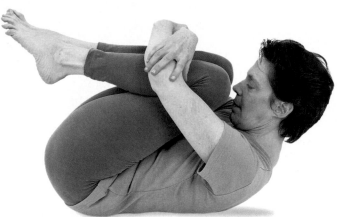

2 Nose to Knees Pose Bend the knees to the chest, wrap the arms around them, and press them tightly to the chest. Bring the head up so that the nose comes as close to the knees as possible. Do Breath of Fire for 2 to 3 minutes. Inhale, stretch. Then exhale and relax down for a few seconds.

4 Spread Stretch Spread the legs as far apart as is comfortable. Inhale and stretch up to the center. Exhale and stretch over the right leg, bringing the forehead toward the knee, and the hands to the toes if possible. Inhale up to the center again, and exhale down to the left leg, reaching the hands toward the toes of the left foot. Continue in this way for 2 to 3 minutes.

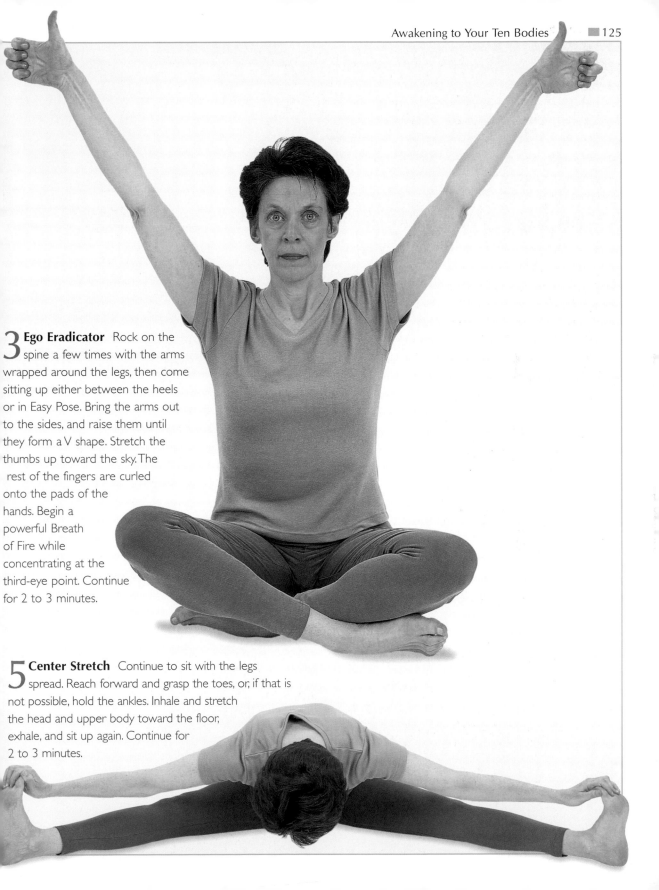

3 Ego Eradicator Rock on the spine a few times with the arms wrapped around the legs, then come sitting up either between the heels or in Easy Pose. Bring the arms out to the sides, and raise them until they form a V shape. Stretch the thumbs up toward the sky. The rest of the fingers are curled onto the pads of the hands. Begin a powerful Breath of Fire while concentrating at the third-eye point. Continue for 2 to 3 minutes.

5 Center Stretch Continue to sit with the legs spread. Reach forward and grasp the toes, or, if that is not possible, hold the ankles. Inhale and stretch the head and upper body toward the floor, exhale, and sit up again. Continue for 2 to 3 minutes.

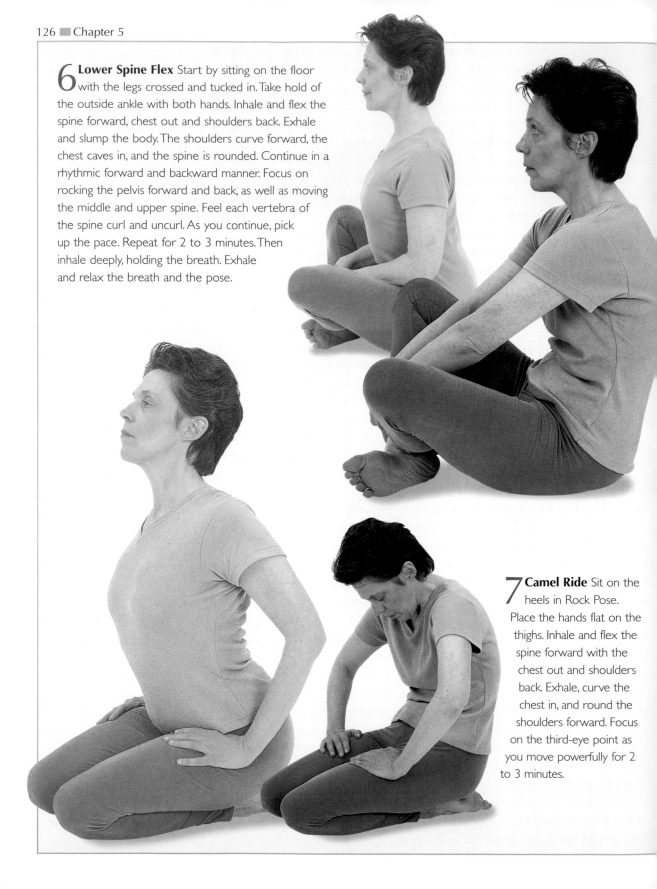

6 **Lower Spine Flex** Start by sitting on the floor with the legs crossed and tucked in. Take hold of the outside ankle with both hands. Inhale and flex the spine forward, chest out and shoulders back. Exhale and slump the body. The shoulders curve forward, the chest caves in, and the spine is rounded. Continue in a rhythmic forward and backward manner. Focus on rocking the pelvis forward and back, as well as moving the middle and upper spine. Feel each vertebra of the spine curl and uncurl. As you continue, pick up the pace. Repeat for 2 to 3 minutes. Then inhale deeply, holding the breath. Exhale and relax the breath and the pose.

7 **Camel Ride** Sit on the heels in Rock Pose. Place the hands flat on the thighs. Inhale and flex the spine forward with the chest out and shoulders back. Exhale, curve the chest in, and round the shoulders forward. Focus on the third-eye point as you move powerfully for 2 to 3 minutes.

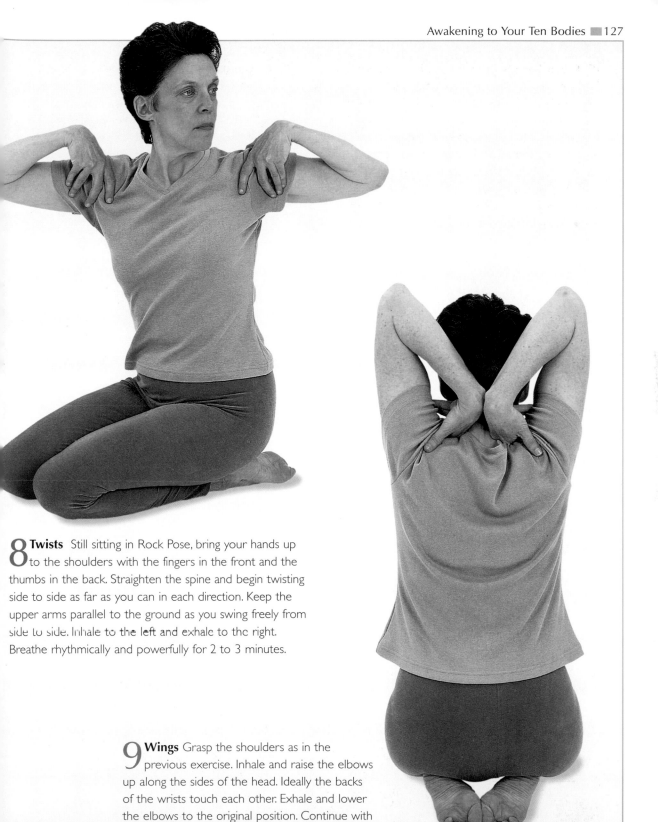

8 Twists Still sitting in Rock Pose, bring your hands up to the shoulders with the fingers in the front and the thumbs in the back. Straighten the spine and begin twisting side to side as far as you can in each direction. Keep the upper arms parallel to the ground as you swing freely from side to side. Inhale to the left and exhale to the right. Breathe rhythmically and powerfully for 2 to 3 minutes.

9 Wings Grasp the shoulders as in the previous exercise. Inhale and raise the elbows up along the sides of the head. Ideally the backs of the wrists touch each other. Exhale and lower the elbows to the original position. Continue with a strong breath for 2 to 3 minutes.

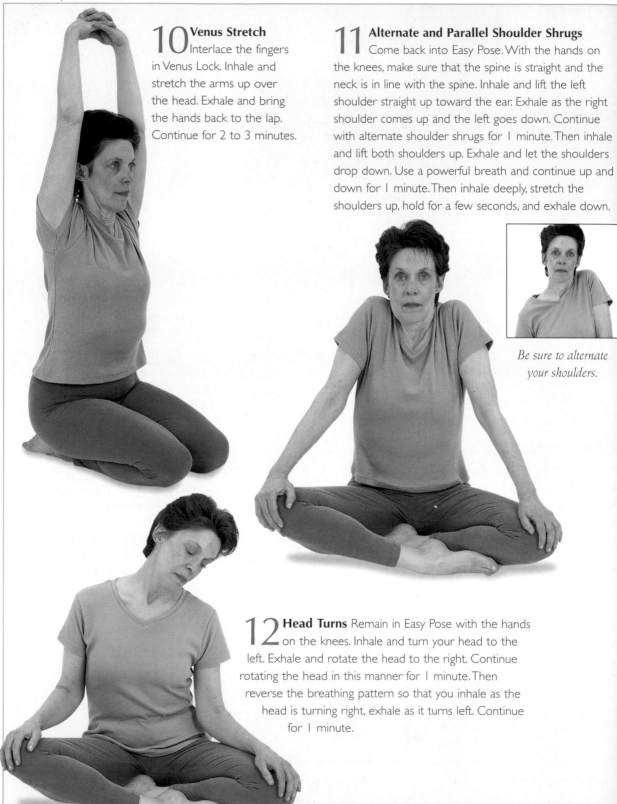

10 Venus Stretch
Interlace the fingers in Venus Lock. Inhale and stretch the arms up over the head. Exhale and bring the hands back to the lap. Continue for 2 to 3 minutes.

11 Alternate and Parallel Shoulder Shrugs
Come back into Easy Pose. With the hands on the knees, make sure that the spine is straight and the neck is in line with the spine. Inhale and lift the left shoulder straight up toward the ear. Exhale as the right shoulder comes up and the left goes down. Continue with alternate shoulder shrugs for 1 minute. Then inhale and lift both shoulders up. Exhale and let the shoulders drop down. Use a powerful breath and continue up and down for 1 minute. Then inhale deeply, stretch the shoulders up, hold for a few seconds, and exhale down.

Be sure to alternate your shoulders.

12 Head Turns Remain in Easy Pose with the hands on the knees. Inhale and turn your head to the left. Exhale and rotate the head to the right. Continue rotating the head in this manner for 1 minute. Then reverse the breathing pattern so that you inhale as the head is turning right, exhale as it turns left. Continue for 1 minute.

13 **Frog Pose** Bring the heels close together and point the toes outward. Squat down with the buttocks close to the heels, the arms between the knees, and the fingers placed on the floor about a foot in front of the feet. The upper body is as straight as possible. Inhale and straighten the legs, bringing the head close to the knees. Exhale and return to the original position. Try to keep the heels slightly off the ground the entire time. Continue for 26 to 54 repetitions, counting 1 inhalation and 1 exhalation as 1 repetition.

14 **Relaxation** Deeply relax on the back for 5 to 10 minutes, then wake the body gently using the wake-up exercises on page 148. Prepare for meditation.

Laya Yoga

This is an example of Laya Yoga, which is a form of meditation that uses rhythmic patterns of mantra and locks. The rhythm of this form easily stays within the subconcious with minimal pracitce. Laya yoga is very powerful and can suspend the mind in a blissful absorption with Infinity.

Sit in Easy Pose with the hands on the knees in *Gian Mudra* (thumb and index finger touching). Chant in a monotone, "*Ek Ong Kar-a, Sat(a) Nam-a, Siri Wha-a Hay Guru*". For each underlined a (pronounced like the u in bus,) in the mantra, pull the Root Lock. The focus is on the navel point pulling inward as the diaphragm is pulled up and the chest lifts. The breath will find its natural rhythm. Visualize the sound spiralling from the base of the spine to the top of the head on each repitition of the mantra. Continue for 11 minutes, increasing to a maximum of 31 minutes. *Ek Ong Kar* translates as "One Creator-Creation." *Sat Nam* means "Truth Manifested," and *Siri Wahe Guru* means "Great Indescribable Wisdom." (See "Resources" for companion CD.)

THREE MINUTES TO ENERGY, CREATIVITY, AND PROSPERITY

The following are simple, quick-acting exercises that can make a difference in just three minutes of practice. They can be practiced together or individually. This kriya is also a good way to take breaks during the day from your usual routine to remind yourself of your higher consciousness.

Energize

Sit in Easy Pose. Bring the arms out to the sides, and raise them until they form a V shape. The fingers are pressing against the mounds of the palms with the thumbs pointing up. Begin Breath of Fire for 3 minutes. Inhale and hold the breath. Quickly begin to make fists of the hands, first with the thumbs inside the fists, then outside. Alternate rapidly as you hold the breath for 15 seconds. Then, with the hands in the original position, slowly bring the thumbs together overhead. Time your movement so that the thumbs meet when you can no longer hold the breath. Slowly lower the arms in an arc around you as you exhale deeply. Sit for 1 minute, breathing slowly.

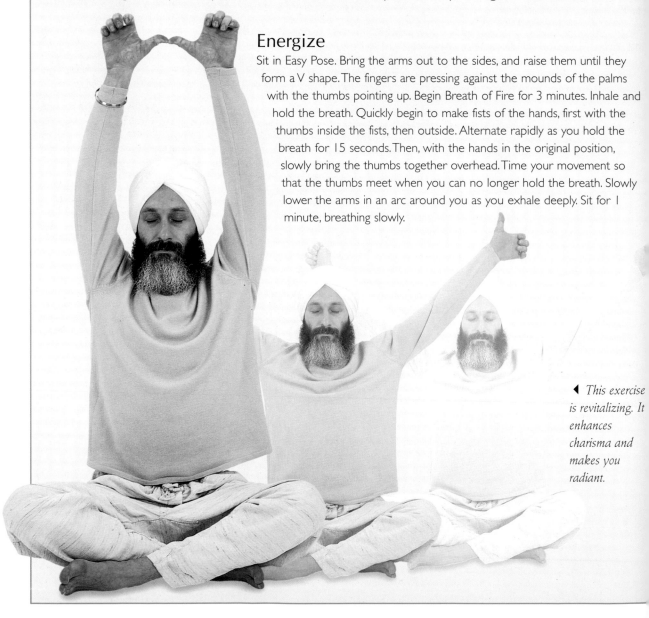

◀ This exercise is revitalizing. It enhances charisma and makes you radiant.

Creativity

Still sitting in Easy Pose, make hands into fists and bring them to the sides of the body at chest level with the elbows pressed back. Extend your chest out. Take 5 deep breaths, then inhale deeply and hold the breath. With the breath held, begin punching the arms alternately. Get mad! When you cannot hold the breath any longer, exhale. Inhale and repeat the powerful punching motion with the held breath. Exhale. Inhale and repeat 1 more time, for a total of 3 times. Then sit, eyes closed, and breathe as slowly as you can for 2 minutes. Stretch and relax.

▶ *This exercise activates the fire in you to spark your creativity.*

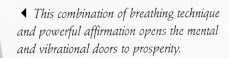

◀ *This combination of breathing technique and powerful affirmation opens the mental and vibrational doors to prosperity.*

Prosperity

Sit in Easy Pose. Keep the spine straight. Look at the center of your chin through your closed eyes, or look at the tip of your nose through partially closed eyes. Inhale deeply and hold, suspending the breath while you mentally recite: "I am bountiful, I am blissful, I am beautiful." Exhale all the breath out, then suspend the breath out as you mentally say "excel, excel, fearless." Practice this for 3 minutes at a time. Feel free to practice 3, 4, or more times a day for 3 minutes each time.

SUBAGH KRIYA
FOR GOOD FORTUNE

Subagh (pronounced "Sue-bog") literally means "fortunate." It is an energetic exercise set to bring spiritual, mental, and material wealth. Yogi Bhajan has said of this kriya, "It's a complete set. . . . If God has written with His own hands that you shall live under misfortune, then by doing Subagh Kriya you can turn your misfortune into prosperity, fortune, and good luck."

This is a five-part kriya. Each part must be practiced for an equal amount of time, either 3 minutes or 11 minutes. Do not exceed 11 minutes for any part. The first exercise may be practiced on its own, separately from the other exercises. (See "Resources" for companion CD.)

1 For Prosperity Sit in Easy Pose with a straight spine. Bend the elbows and bring the palms up in front of the chest, facing in toward the chest. Strike the outer sides of the hands together, forcefully hitting the area from the base of the little finger to the base of the palm. Then turn the hands so that the backs of the hands are facing you as they hit along the length of the index fingers. The thumbs will naturally move slightly away so the index fingers can hit. Hit hard! Alternately strike the outside edge of the hands, then the inside. As they strike, chant *Har* (the Infinite One). Chant with the tip of the tongue touching the roof of the mouth as you roll the *r* and pulling the navel in on each repetition of *Har*. Your eyes are slightly open and focused at the tip of the nose in a soft gaze.

This exercise/meditation can be done on its own to increase prosperity. The sound Har *embodies the "green" energy of money. It has been said that this exercise is a "money-making machine," in the sense that it can help you open to the infinite flow of abundance. Hitting the sides of the hands activates meridians that access brainpower.*

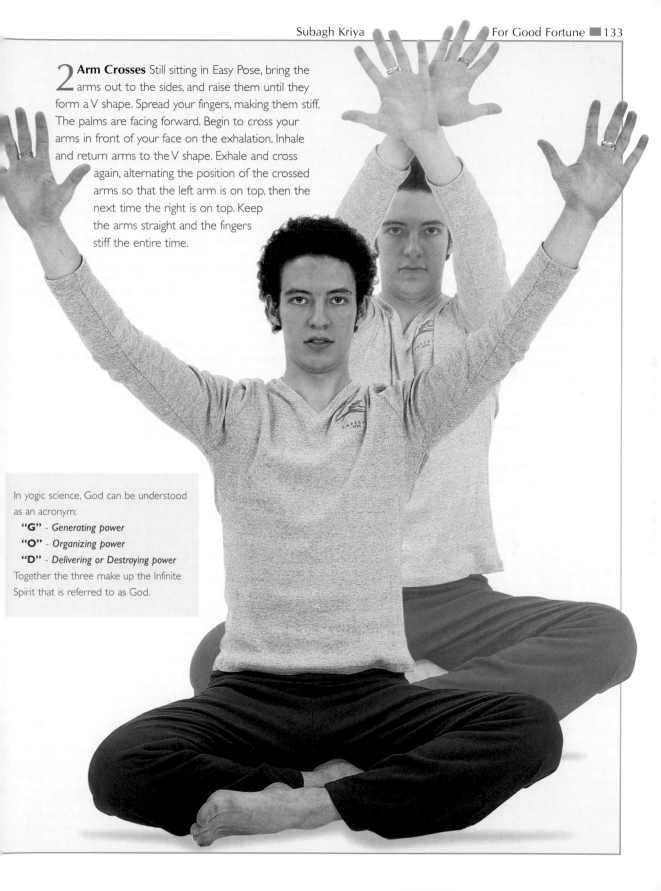

2 **Arm Crosses** Still sitting in Easy Pose, bring the arms out to the sides, and raise them until they form a V shape. Spread your fingers, making them stiff. The palms are facing forward. Begin to cross your arms in front of your face on the exhalation. Inhale and return arms to the V shape. Exhale and cross again, alternating the position of the crossed arms so that the left arm is on top, then the next time the right is on top. Keep the arms straight and the fingers stiff the entire time.

In yogic science, God can be understood as an acronym:

"G" - *Generating power*

"O" - *Organizing power*

"D" - *Delivering or Destroying power*

Together the three make up the Infinite Spirit that is referred to as God.

3 **Backward Circles** Still with the
arms raised in a V shape, make a fist
around your thumb, squeezing your thumb
tightly as if you are trying to squeeze all the blood
out of it. Keeping the arms up and straight, move the
arms in small backward circles, continuing to squeeze the
thumbs. Begin to chant the mantra God powerfully from
your navel. Each time you make 1 backward circle, chant 1
repetition of the mantra. Move powerfully, so that the entire
spine shakes. You may even lift off the ground slightly by the
strong movement.

4 **Chopping Motion** Still sitting in Easy Pose, bend your elbows with
your forearms parallel to the ground. The hands are at the level of
the diaphragm and the palms are flat, facing the body. (One palm–it does
not matter which - should be closer to your body with the other behind
it.) Begin to move the left hand down a few inches as the right hand
moves up a few inches. Then switch. Continue moving the hands up
and down between the heart and navel in a smooth motion.

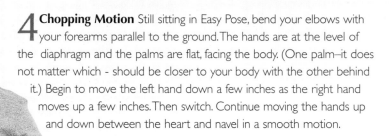

Coordinate the movement with the following chant: *Har, Haray, Haree,
Wahe Guru.* Remember to touch the roof of the mouth on the r
sounds, softly rolling them. Remember to pronounce *Guru* as "G'roo,"
softly rolling the *r*. Chant in a monotone with 1 repetition of the
mantra approximately every 4 seconds. Chant in the following way:
For 3 minutes total, chant out loud for 1 minute, whisper strongly for
1 minute, then whistle (mentally repeating the sound) for 1
minute. If you are doing this exercise for 11 minutes, chant out
loud for 6 minutes, whisper for 3 minutes, then whistle for 2.
The first part of the mantra gives different aspects of *Har,*
the Infinite Being. The second part of the mantra, *Wahe Guru,*
expresses the happiness of merger with *Har.* (See "Resources"
for companion CD.)

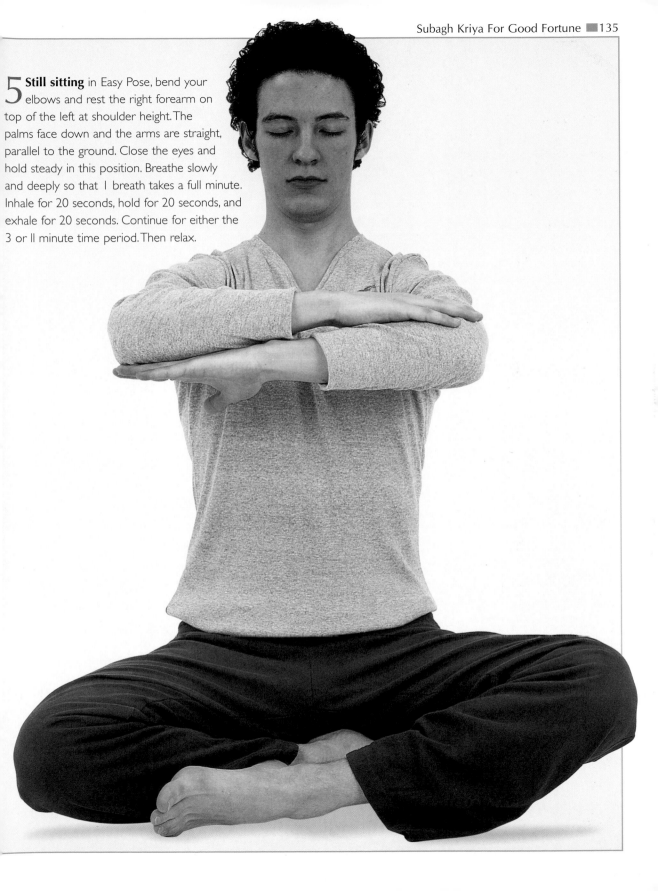

5 Still sitting in Easy Pose, bend your elbows and rest the right forearm on top of the left at shoulder height. The palms face down and the arms are straight, parallel to the ground. Close the eyes and hold steady in this position. Breathe slowly and deeply so that 1 breath takes a full minute. Inhale for 20 seconds, hold for 20 seconds, and exhale for 20 seconds. Continue for either the 3 or 11 minute time period. Then relax.

KRIYA FOR
ONENESS

For years and years we have created such fear. What we have done is we have separated ourselves from God; "He's in the seventh heavens, we are down here." No, like the rays of the sun which shine, all of you have come here, you are part of the same Reality, same Truth, same Grace...If you simply understand and write on your heart, **"Made In God,"** *all your problems will be over.*

–Yogi Bhajan

*Visualize the oneness. Visualize, visualize.
See the union happening.*

–Yogi Bhajan

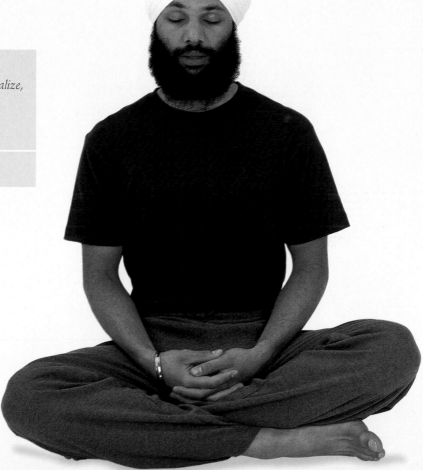

1 **God and Me** Sit with a straight spine in Easy Pose. Interlace your hands together in your lap. Close the eyes and sing the affirmation, "God and me, me and God, are One." Start softly, and slowly begin chanting louder and louder. Continue for 3 minutes, then inhale deeply, exhale, and immediately begin the next exercise.

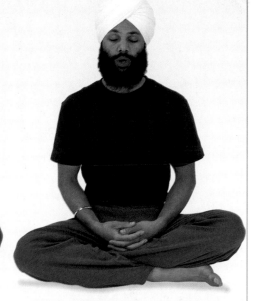

Burn out the fire inside with breath of fire. Fast, fast . . . Use your diaphragm and your navel point. Become the strength of the day . . . You know if there's a glow on your face and your personality is smiling, you're walking tall and you have all the strength, hundreds of people will love you. If you're a brick-face, do not talk, do not look and see into the eyes of somebody; what are you going to be, a dead rat? Come on! Breathe! Energize your being.

–Yogi Bhajan

2 **Breath of Fire** Still sitting in Easy Pose, bring your interlaced hands onto the navel center and begin a strong Breath of Fire. Move the diaphragm powerfully and press on the navel. Move so that your shoulders jump like you are dancing. Move fast and with great force. Continue for 2 minutes.

3 **Circle Breath** Still sitting in Easy Pose, hands interlaced in the lap, make your mouth into a circle and begin breathing in and out through the mouth. Breathe quickly and powerfully for 1 minute. Go immediately on to the next exercise.

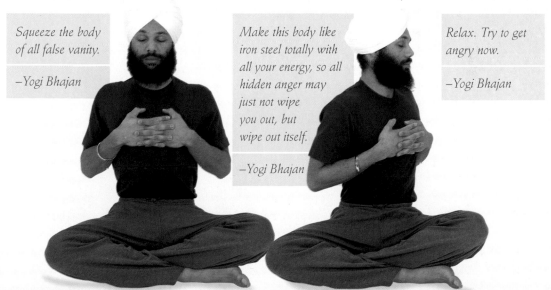

Squeeze the body of all false vanity.

–Yogi Bhajan

Make this body like iron steel totally with all your energy, so all hidden anger may just not wipe you out, but wipe out itself.

–Yogi Bhajan

Relax. Try to get angry now.

–Yogi Bhajan

4 **Iron Steel Body** Inhale deeply. Hold the breath tight and lock your hands, pressing them against the heart center. Then exhale. Breathe in again deeply and hold. Exhale. Now breathe in deep and hold. Turn left tightly, and turn right tightly. Come to the center and hold yourself as tightly as you possibly can. Hold the breath as long as you possibly can. Then exhale, relaxing the posture.

TO BE RID OF
INTERNAL ANGER

This kriya is designed to forcefully remove internal anger that would normally take years to eliminate.

You can judge it for yourself. If you do this for a few days the very internal anger for which you are suffering, and which is coming from the subconscious in many ways through your personality, will disappear. That inner anger has to come out. It has to find a way. Why don't you volunteer yourself and get it out? Why to suffer? This is a very powerful exercise, and afterward you get into a state of ecstasy . . . Once your inner anger is out, all you are left with is wisdom.

—Yogi Bhajan

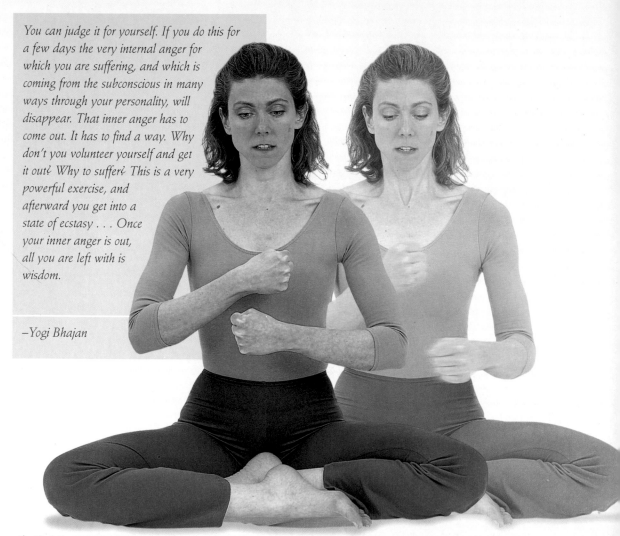

1 Fighting Pose Sit with a straight spine. Bring your hands into tight fists and begin to "hit" the space between the hands at the solar plexus area. The forearms will cross each other at chest level. As they cross with a force, powerfully chant the mantra *Har* (The Infinite One). Remember to pull the navel in as you chant, and strike the tongue on the roof of the mouth on the rolled *r*. Keep up the striking motion with the fists. Hit hard so that the whole body reverberates. Chant powerfully. Continue for 7 minutes. Then inhale deeply. Make the hands tight like iron rods in front of your chest. Hold for 10 to 15 seconds, then exhale. Repeat 2 more times for a total of 3. Make your hands completely stiff as you hold each inhale. Then relax.

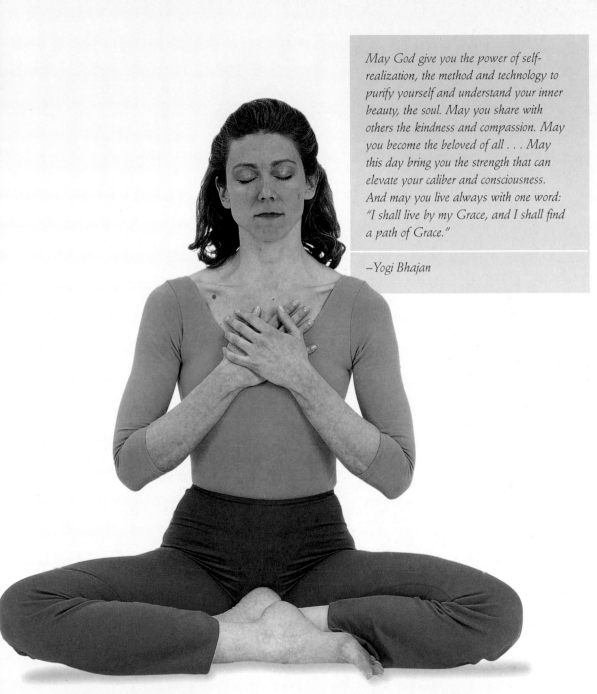

May God give you the power of self-realization, the method and technology to purify yourself and understand your inner beauty, the soul. May you share with others the kindness and compassion. May you become the beloved of all . . . May this day bring you the strength that can elevate your caliber and consciousness. And may you live always with one word: "I shall live by my Grace, and I shall find a path of Grace."

—Yogi Bhajan

2 Calm Meditation Sit with a straight spine. Close your eyes. Bring both hands to the heart center, one on top of the other. Go into a deep, calm meditation. Trust, feel, and imagine nonexistence. Just let yourself go. The power released is being replaced by the self, the neutral self. It will balance out your energy. Continue for 8 minutes. Inhale, exhale, and relax.

FOR HEART, SHOULDERS, AND CIRCULATION

This kriya focuses on releasing tightness in the shoulders, increasing circulation—especially in the breast/lung area—and strengthening the heart chakra. Each of the first three exercises uses the strong "O" breath, inhaling and exhaling through the circled mouth. There is no break between exercises. The fourth exercise uses drum music from India, which you can order from one of the organizations in the Resources section, or substitute with other uplifting drum music.

▶ *This exercise builds your stamina and rejuvenates the nervous system. It relaxes the body inside out, takes away your muscle fatigue, and makes you steady. It strengthens the heart center, and helps to break up locked areas in the lungs. The movement was described by Yogi Bhajan in the following way: "[This exercise] is a very electromagnetic field system. You are neutral [as you touch the two hands together]. Then the 1, 2, 3 [inhaling breath] power. Then you touch the earth, pick up the negative [earth's magnetic pull], and you are done. Simple."*

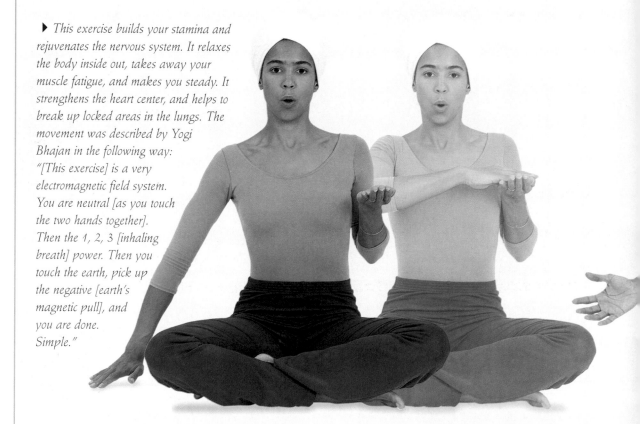

1 **For the Heart Chakra** Sit straight in Easy Pose. Bend the left elbow and bring the left hand up to the heart level, with the palm facing forward. The left palm is open and relaxed. The right hand will touch the ground on the right side of you, then arc up and touch the left hand, palm to palm. This motion is continued with the following breathing pattern: When the right hand moves from the left hand back to the floor, take

3 inhalations through the circled mouth. As the right hand moves back from the floor to the left hand, exhale in 1 strong exhale from the circled mouth. The 3 inhalations are almost like sips of air, and the exhalation is a blowing-out motion. Use the diaphragm to help you breathe powerfully. Continue for 4 minutes, then close the eyes and increase the speed of the motion. Continue for another 4 minutes.

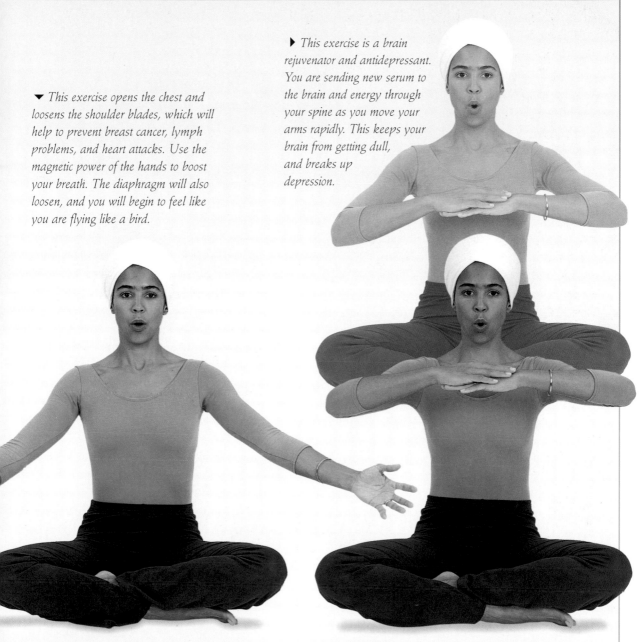

▼ *This exercise opens the chest and loosens the shoulder blades, which will help to prevent breast cancer, lymph problems, and heart attacks. Use the magnetic power of the hands to boost your breath. The diaphragm will also loosen, and you will begin to feel like you are flying like a bird.*

▶ *This exercise is a brain rejuvenator and antidepressant. You are sending new serum to the brain and energy through your spine as you move your arms rapidly. This keeps your brain from getting dull, and breaks up depression.*

2 Fly Like a Bird Still sitting in Easy Pose, bring the arms out in front and slightly to the sides. Begin to make large backward circles with the two arms, coordinating the circles so that both arms circle inward and outward together. The hands are relaxed and facing forward. The circles are about 30 inches in diameter. Use the O breath through the mouth, in rhythm with the arm movement. Move and breathe powerfully. Continue for 3½ minutes.

3 Arm Flutters Still sitting in Easy Pose, bend the elbows and extend them out to the sides, at shoulder level. Bring the hands in front of the heart center, palms down with the right palm flat on top of the back of the left hand. Begin to raise the hands up a few inches and down a few inches from the heart center, very rapidly, in a fluttering motion. Keep the elbows out to the sides, and move the forearms. Breathe through the "O" mouth powerfully and rhythmically.

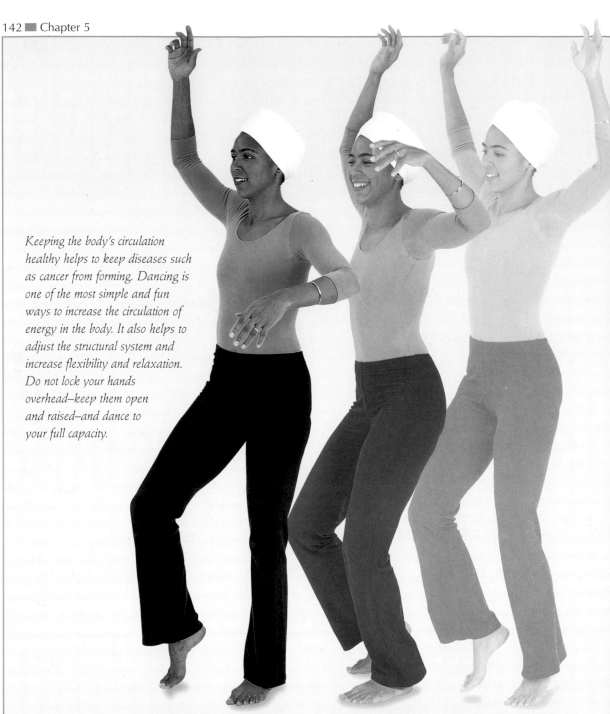

Keeping the body's circulation healthy helps to keep diseases such as cancer from forming. Dancing is one of the most simple and fun ways to increase the circulation of energy in the body. It also helps to adjust the structural system and increase flexibility and relaxation. Do not lock your hands overhead–keep them open and raised–and dance to your full capacity.

4 **Dance with Drums** Immediately stand up and begin to dance to drum music. When this yoga set was originally given, this exercise was accompanied by Bangara Rhythms and Punjabi drums. Lift and move your shoulders as you dance. Open the shoulder area. You must dance powerfully to break up the blocks in the body and adjust the spine and neck. Continue for 6 minutes. (See "Resources" for music.) Then continue to dance, and focus on keeping your arms up, moving them as you dance. Move the hands and hips in balance. Keep the hands up to open you shoulders and ribcage. Allow yourself to sweat. Continue another 6 minutes.

▼ *This opens up your lower back, and affects the part of the lower back that is hard to release even through massage. It can adjust the lower back so that it will release and open as much as a few inches.*

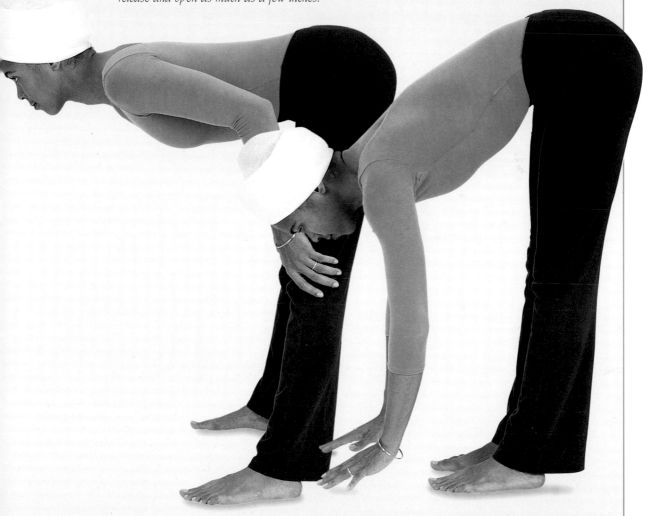

5 Deep Stretch Straddle your legs about 3 feet apart. Keep the legs straight but not locked. Put the hands on the knees and bend forward so that your back is parallel to the ground. Hold and breathe normally. Make your body into the shape of the number 7.

6 Stretch and Bounce Bend forward, touch the ground with your hands, then bounce up and down. Slowly and gradually stretch out the lower back. Let your hands and arms stretch toward the floor as you bounce. Continue for 45 seconds. Then inhale deeply when bent over, exhale strongly and stand up. Repeat 4 more times, inhaling down, exhaling up. Then relax.

CHAPTER 6

THE ART OF
DEEP
RELAXATION

"When your self is in peace, then all the
surroundings shall be in peace."
–*Yogi Bhajan*

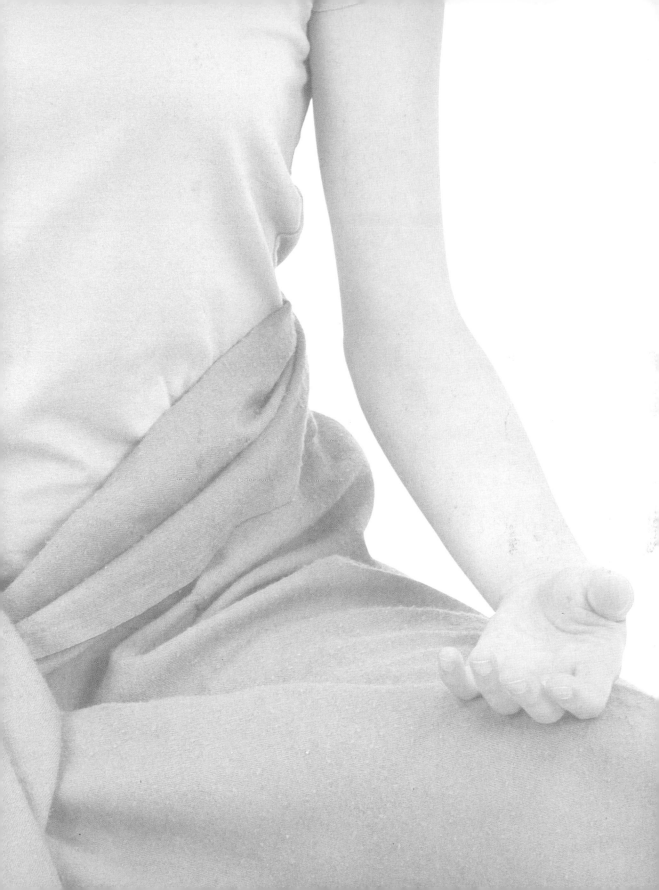

RELAXATION IN YOUR
YOGA PRACTICE

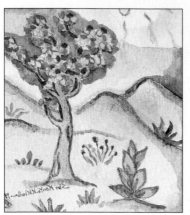

The effects of the kriyas in this book will be greatly enhanced by practicing relaxation at the end of each kriya. Seemingly passive, the deep relaxation after a yoga set is decidedly active. During deep relaxation, many biochemical and energetic changes take place as the effects of the kriya are assimilated within the psyche and body. It is most important to give the space for these changes to take place. By setting aside time for deep relaxation, you are affirming a trust in the innate wisdom of the body to self-heal and regenerate.

A meditative mind and a relaxed mind go together. Your relaxation practice will enhance your meditation, and the practice of meditation will teach you to relax. The natural flow of a practice of Kundalini Yoga followed by deep relaxation and ending with meditation, will give the perfect energy balance to the body and mind.

Beginning the path to relaxation is beginning the path of awareness. Do not be discouraged to find tension in your body as you begin to practice relaxing deeply. Awareness is the first step. You are relearning how to process tension, which is your body's natural reaction to stressful situations. Ask yourself, where is my body feeling tense? What is my breath doing? Stress, which depletes our reservoirs of energy, also speeds up our metabolism to the point that even when we do have a chance to slow down, we find ourselves unable to unwind and relax. The good news is that even if the actual stressful situation cannot be changed, reducing the body's reaction to stress by practicing "on the spot" relaxation can help the mind and body break the stress cycle, and learn to relax. As your yoga practice deepens, you become more aware of tension in your body and mind, and are able to consciously relax yourself immediately. This ability to relax eventually carries over into your daily life.

Practicing "on the spot" relaxation can be done in a number of ways, depending on which appeals to you most. The essential ingredient in this recipe for dealing with stress is the breath. In a stressful situation, you may want to excuse yourself, go to a private place, and take ten long and deep breaths with the eyes closed. Be aware of tension forming in the body, and consciously relax it, much in the same way you do when you are practicing a deep stretch in your yoga routine. Use visualizations that work for you. Some of the tools of stress release include: visualizing the prana, or light-energy, filling you on the inhalation; feeling the stress leaving on the exhalation; and focusing on mantra and affirmations on the breath.

HOW TO PRACTICE
DEEP RELAXATION

The deep relaxation practice that takes place at the end of each yoga set in Kundalini Yoga gives you a deeply peaceful experience to carry over into the rest of your life.

- Have a natural fabric mat underneath your body, and a light natural fabric shawl to cover yourself with. If you are wearing glasses, take them off at this time to relax the eyes. Have some beautifully uplifting music playing softly. The words should be elevating and divinely inspired. Mantras and affirmations are recommended (see "Resources" for companion CD).

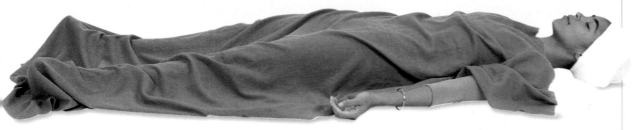

- Lie down on the back in Corpse Pose, so named because it provides the opportunity to become "dead" to the old and prepare the way for a new consciousness. Corpse Pose is done by putting the arms down at the sides with the palms relaxed and facing upward. Allow the fingers to curl naturally. Allow the legs to relax and fall slightly outward. If the lower back is sensitive in this position, place a rolled towel or small pillow under the knees. Close the eyes. Relax the lips, tongue, jaws, and face muscles. Allow the mouth to feel as if you are about to smile. Allow the body to feel as if it is sinking toward the floor.
- Close the eyes, and let the mind follow the breath. Mentally scan the body, starting with the feet and moving upward slowly. Visualize and feel the inhalation bringing light and energy (prana) to each part. On the exhalation, visualize and feel tension releasing from each part. You may prefer to do this slowly, paying attention to detail, or to mentally sweep over the body moderately fast.
- Notice your mind. If it begins to wander, bring your attention back to quiet inflow and outflow of the breath. If you like, you can hear the mantra *Sat Nam* as you inhale and exhale. If your mind starts to wander into the past or future, bring your attention back to the breath.
- Bless yourself. Dwell in your innermost heart. Expand into the universal consciousness. Do so in whatever way speaks to you.
- Continue to relax for at least 5 minutes, preferably longer. If you go into a sleep, it will not be the same kind of sleep you usually have. It is a self-healing sleep, so light that you may feel yourself almost dancing on the edge of awareness.

COMING BACK AFTER RELAXATION

At the end of the relaxation time, when you come back to awareness of yourself, take a deep and conscious inhale and exhale. Do the following wake-up exercises for about 30 seconds each, using deep breathing.

▼ *All 72,000 nerve endings in the feet and hands are stimulated and the electromagnetic energy field is rebalanced. Palming the eyes relaxes and heals the eyes, which process much of our sensory information.*

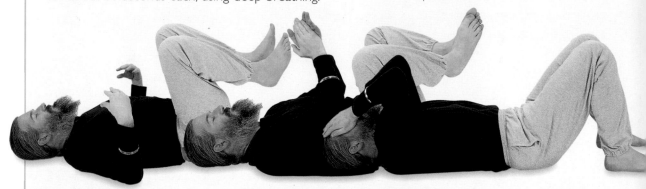

Roll your wrists and ankles in circles in both directions. This awakens the extremities of the body.

Pick up your feet and begin to rub the soles of your feet together (preferably, with bare feet). At the same time, rub your hands together. Put the feet down after a time while continuing to rub the hands until they are very warm.

Then place the palms over the eyes and send the relaxing warmth into the eyes. Breathe deeply and relax the entire face.

Cat Stretch: Bring your arms out to the sides. Lift one bent leg and bring it across the other in a diagonal stretch. Breathe. Then switch sides. Do this a few times on each side.

This exercise gives a good diagonal stretch to the entire body and spine. Draw your knees into your chest and wrap the arms around them. Tuck your head into your knees and begin rocking up and down on your spine 6 to 8 times.

▶ *Anytime the body has been sleeping or resting deeply, these exercises will bring the body and mind to consciousness gently and completely. Be sure to drink some purified water (at room temperature) after relaxing, or meditating to reground and rebalance the nervous system.*

This energizes the spine. Sit up to end your practice or to meditate.

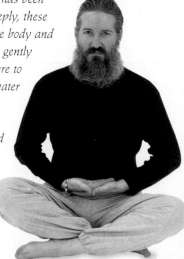

MENTAL RELAXATION

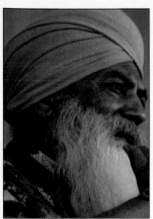

The following relaxation is given by Yogi Bhajan in his own words. Lie down in Corpse Pose and have someone read to you slowly, or play back a recording of your own voice repeating this mental relaxation. Hearing yourself in this way is healing and uplifiting.

"Relax in total existence, relating under the total ordinance of your higher consciousness. Each cell of your body must relax. You are going to be a totally, extremely relaxed individual. Absolutely relax, relax with dignity, with perfect heart and consciousness, with sweetness and beauty. Feel every cell of your body relaxing, deeper and deeper, steadier and steadier, and steadier and steadier. Survey yourself in any form and self-situation. Let everything go. Let all the tension go. When you relax your body, God will prevail because the prana will prevail. It is the prevailing of the prana that gives you absolute health. Oh dear one, just relax, feel that the fingertips are falling away, the wrists are going away, everything is breaking. Shatter your body into all its cells. Build it up. Vibrate your tattvas* into tattvas. Let your mind collaborate with you at this moment. Relax your body, your eyes, your eyebrows, your cheeks, your chin, your neck, your head, shoulders, rib cage, belly, and everything in it, waistline, thighs, shins, ankles, feet, toes—everything. Let the Divine flow through you. Let you receive it. Every part of it is yours. It is your privilege and you must have that privilege. Be extremely relaxed, and use your mind to relax yourself. One who cannot relax himself on command has not known his command yet. It is the highest power of the self; therefore, please command yourself to relax. Become the master of the self. Let this physical self obey your mental self, and the prana, the soul, must prevail through you."

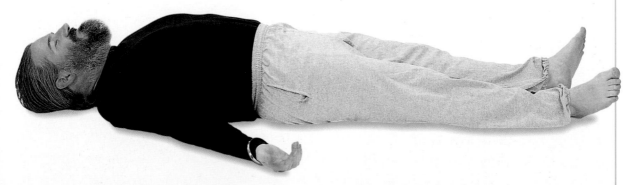

* Tattvas (Tut/vaas): *The five elements of which everything is composed: fire, air, earth, ether, and water.*

THE ANCIENT GONG

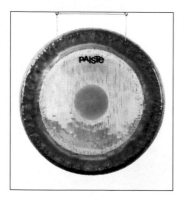

(In "Resources," see companion CD for the sound of the Gong.)

For countless centuries, the gong has been used as a consciousness-transforming tool. Today, with the increased understanding of how sound affects the human, the power of the gong is beginning to be recognized in scientific circles. In the yogic science, the sound of the gong can repattern the gray matter of the brain, help eliminate diseased cells in the body, and balance the chakras. Many people have experienced profound transformation, self-healing, and a state of peaceful awareness through the gong's vibration, either in deep relaxation or through sitting in meditation.

How to Relax With the Gong Lie down on the back in Corpse Pose. Cover with a light, natural blanket or shawl. Take some long, deep breaths and relax. Let the sound of the gong penetrate every cell of your being. In the process of listening to the gong, your mind may move through different stages. You may feel yourself opening to the expansive, freeing sound, then wanting to resist and close at other stages of the playing of the gong. If intense feelings begin to surface, remember to breathe consciously. Everything can be allowed, and once allowed, will pass through your awareness, cleansing the mind. The gong will facilitate your passing through resistance and fear. Let yourself be washed in the waves of the gong for 5 to 11 minutes or more. Be sure to bring yourself back by breathing deeply, and doing the wake-up exercises. You may like to extend your relaxation by listening to some beautiful, uplifting music after the gong.

Using the Gong in Meditation Sit with a straight spine, hands relaxed in whatever mudra feels comfortable. Allow the sound to penetrate your body and mind. Sit and breathe for 5 to 11 minutes or more. Inhale, exhale, and stretch your body to end.

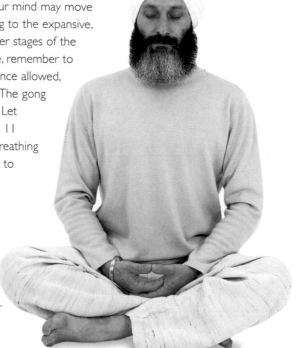

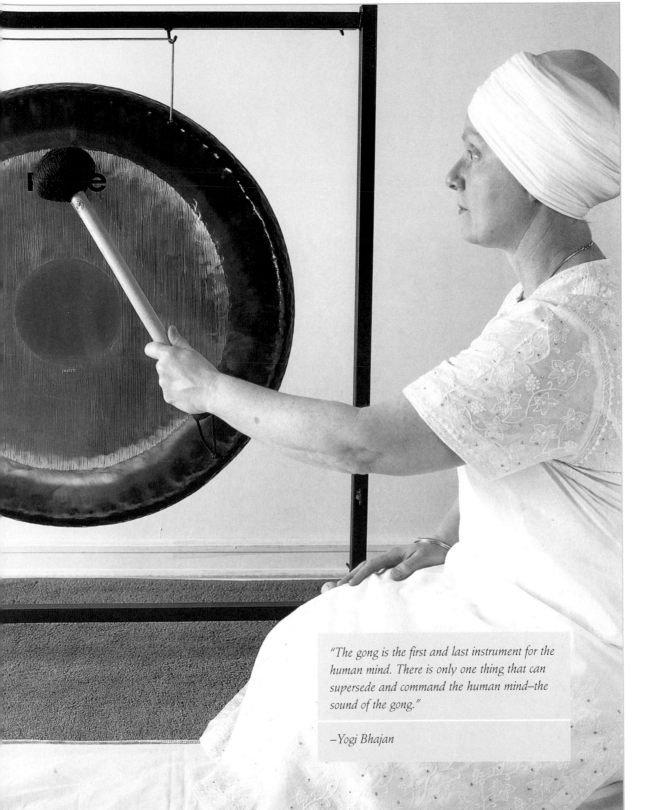

"The gong is the first and last instrument for the human mind. There is only one thing that can supersede and command the human mind–the sound of the gong."

–Yogi Bhajan

CHAPTER 7

MEDITATION

"Prayer is when the mind is one-pointed
and man talks to Infinity. Meditation is
when the mind becomes totally clean and
receptive, and Infinity talks to man."

–Yogi Bhajan

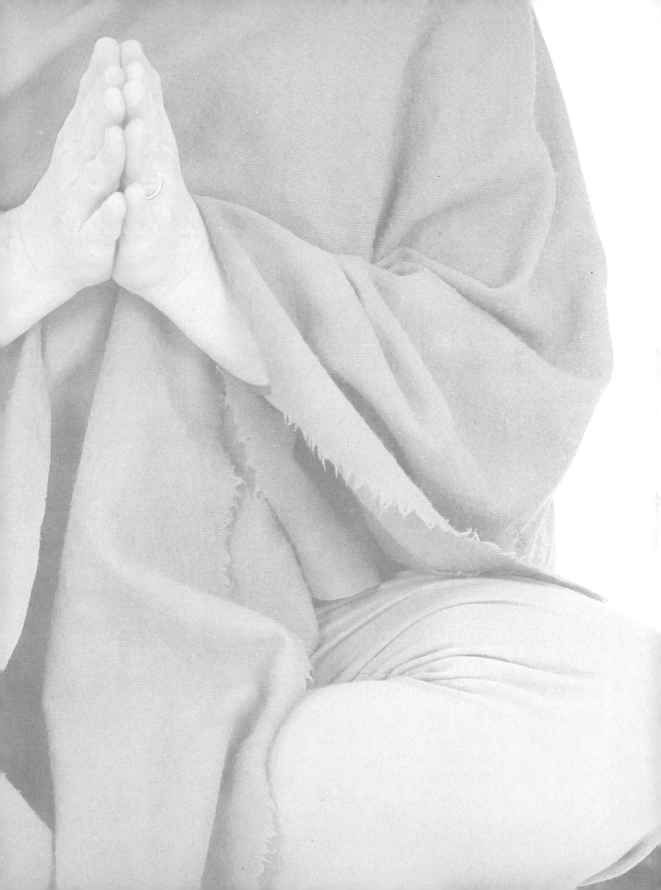

UNDERSTANDING
MEDITATION

Practicing Kundalini Yoga is one of the best ways to prepare yourself for meditation. The meditative focus on the breath is basic to Kundalini Yoga. As you exercise and move your body, your concentration is on the rhythmic breathing patterns. After a time of regular Kundalini Yoga practice, using a silent mantra on the breath, usually *Sat Nam*, becomes second nature. When you sit for the purpose of meditation, you take this one step further by stilling the body and focusing solely on meditating deeply. The skills you learn from Kundalini Yoga, focusing on the breath and using mantra, are invaluable in the process of meditation.

The yogis developed their minds to be their servant, not their master. They did this through meditation. First the body must be stilled. In that stillness, the mind will begin to jump about. At this point, the yogic practices of proper posture, inner concentration, and focus on the breath and/or mantra are essential. A person who has the patience to allow the mind to go through whatever antics it will, while remaining firmly planted, will experience something. That "something" is different for each one, but it will be, in some way or another, a reawakening of the self. With this new awareness comes inner change, then outer change. Through the meditative mind, the human takes his or her rightful place as the master of the house.

By simply letting thoughts pass by, and not dumping them into the subconscious mind, where they can resurface at any emotional trigger, the mind is cleansed. The person is literally renewed. Once your mind starts becoming used to this process, meditation becomes very cozy, very heartful. You will want to do it again and again. In the beginning, you may not be able to do it for very long. Gradually, as you develop that coziness, this initial barrage of thoughts becomes shorter and shorter. After a time of practice, you will find your meditative mind responding instantly to your call. Eventually, you can remain in an elevated consciousness for much of your daily life.

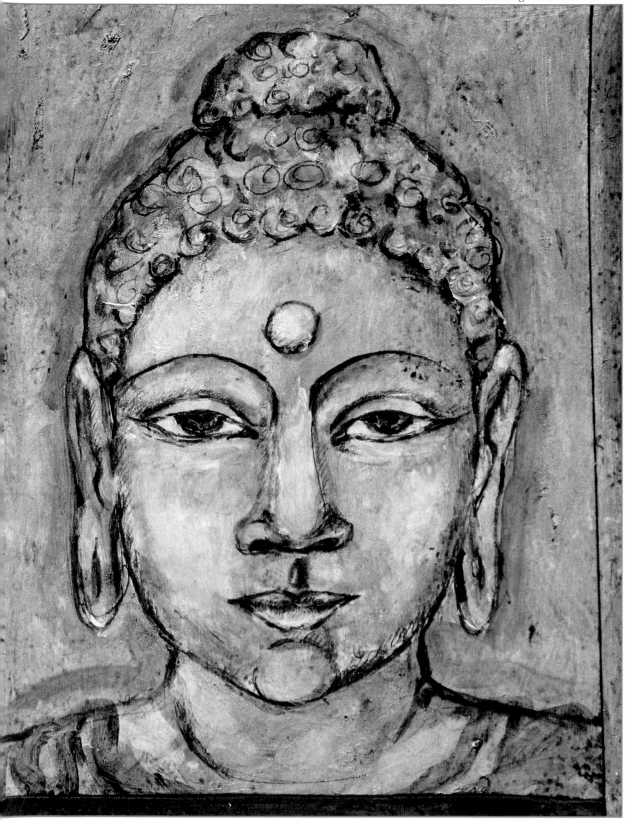

ELEMENTS OF
MEDITATION

POSTURE

The most important element in sitting for meditation is the position of the spine. You may sit in any of the given postures as long as the spine is straight: Easy Pose, Lotus, or on a chair, . A straight spine will allow the kundalini energy to flow without restriction. Adjust your posture by closing the eyes and feeling how well the vertebra of the spine, including the cervical vertebra, are lined up.

BREATH

Most meditations given in this book will specify a type of breathing pattern. If none is provided, allow the breath to come in and out naturally. Breathing deeply and consciously will affect you both physically (by circulating oxygen and pranic energy to all body systems) and psychologically (by bringing the mind to rest in the present moment.)

MENTAL FOCUS

Besides the most common focal points of the third-eye point and the heart center, many meditations also give instructions for other points of concentration. A common one is to focus on the tip of the nose, usually with the eyes slightly open. Generally, when a meditation specifies open eyes, your gaze should be soft, and eyes almost closed. Another focal point in meditation is the top of the skull, which is also referred to as the crown chakra or Tenth Gate. For gazing upward at the crown, and to some degree, the third eye, gently turn the closed eyes upward to "view" through those higher centers. If this is too difficult at first, you can "feel" those centers without pressing the eyes upward.

Why Different Focal Points?

Beaming your mind's "light" on the different chakras during meditation produces different effects. Following is a summary of the different focal points and the regions they affect.

• Crown: Elevates one into higher consciousness and activates the pineal gland, which controls the nucleus projection of every cell of the body.
• Third-eye: Stimulates the pituitary gland, the master gland for the glandular system. Activates the intuition, the ability to know the unknown.

• Tip of the nose: Steadies then locks the mind into the meditation. New energy pathways are created in the brain patterns.
• The Moon Center (chin): Mentally looking out through the chin allows one to see oneself clearly.

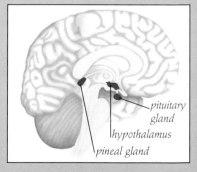

Master glands

MANTRA

Many meditations focus on a silent or chanted mantra. In some meditations, the instructions are to chant in a monotone. Generally, this type of chanting focuses the mind and changes brain patterns. Other meditations have mantras that are sung. Singing opens the heart center and the pranic body.

Affirmations are positive statements that, when spoken, retrain the mind. Many times they will be in one's own language.

A common belief is that in meditation, one does not think. According to yogic teachings, the mind releases a thousand thoughts per wink of the eye! We choose certain thoughts to pay attention to and many others pass through unnoticed. When you sit down to meditate, and your awareness turns inward, you may notice this steady stream of thoughts. If you beam that light of awareness on one thought, the others will recede into the background and pass through without being energized by your attention.

> "Typically, we dissipate our mental energy. It spreads out in all directions at once like the light from a bulb. But with a mantra, the mind's energy can focus. When the energy of a single bulb is focused with a crystal in a particular way, it becomes a laser capable of even cutting steel. In the same way, when you focus your mental energy with a mantra, it becomes incredibly potent."
>
> –Subagh Singh Khalsa
> Meditation for Absolutely Everyone

The mantra is a consciously chosen thought. By substituting the mantra for other thoughts, there simply is no room for other thoughts. The mantra contains the sound vibration to elevate you. By chanting or repeating a mantra, the meridian points on the upper palate are stimulated, the hypothalamus secretes, and the chemistry of the upper centers of the brain are transformed. This is the scientific process of being in "higher consciousness."

MEDITATION TIME

Yogic science has determined that there are specific amounts of "processing" time needed to create certain desired effects during meditation. Practitioners of Kundalini Yoga are encouraged to start modestly and increase slowly to the longer times given for meditation. (Most meditations are done for 11 or 31 minutes.)

---

3 minutes:
Your circulation and blood stability is affected.

11 minutes:
The pituitary and nerves begin to change.

22 minutes:
The three minds (Negative, Positive, and Neutral) balance and begin to work together.

31 minutes:
Meditation begins to affect your whole mind, your aura, and all your body's internal elements (the tattvas: earth, air, ether, water, fire).

62 minutes:
Your subconscious "shadow mind" and your positive (outer) projection are integrated.

2½ hours:
Holds the change in the subconscious mind throughout the cycle of the day.

PERIODS OF TIME TO AFFECT CHANGES

In much the same way that there are specific amounts of time for practicing meditation, there are specific cycles of time that help change old habits and develop new ones. Often a practitioner of Kundalini Yoga and meditation chooses a specific kriya or meditation that works on the body and mind to affect a desired change. He or she then commits to a program of doing the chosen kriya/meditation for 40, 90, 120, or sometimes 1,000 days. Each amount of time will give specific results:

---

40 days:
It takes 40 days to change a habit.

90 days:
It takes 90 days to confirm the habit.

120 days:
The new habit is who you are.

1,000 days:
You have mastered the new habit.

SPECIFIC
MEDITATIONS

BEGINNER'S MEDITATION

Sit in Easy Pose. Make sure that the spine is straight by mentally following the spine from the base to the neck. A firm pillow may be used under the buttocks to help straighten the lower spine and relax the hips downward. Close the eyes. Begin to follow your breath coming in and going out. Be aware of expanding the abdomen on the inhalation and emptying it on the exhalation. Allow the chest to expand as the breath travels upward on the inhalation. Feel the chest relax downward on the exhalation.

After a short time of feeling the breath, begin to place your attention at your heart center as you inhale and exhale. If you like, you can begin to hear the sound of *Sat* as you inhale, and *Nam* as you exhale. Or you can hear "I am" on the inhalation, and "I am" on the exhalation

After a short time, while keeping an awareness of the third-eyepoint, add in an awareness of the heart center again. Feel both at the same time. Notice what that feels like for you. You may have a sensation that light is beaming from your heart and mind. Or you may feel peace and calm, or love coming from these centers. You may experience something entirely different. Everyone's experience is unique, and just right for them.

Now begin to move your awareness from the heart center to the third-eye point. Without straining, feel yourself residing at the place between your eyebrows. You may gently turn your eyes upward to do this, if you like. The important thing is that there is no strain. Keep your face relaxed. Again, you may put a mantra or affirmation on the breath as you inhale and exhale consciously.

Continue "playing" with this meditation for as long as you like. When you are finished, inhale deeply and stretch your spine up and your arms overhead, shaking them vigorously for 10 seconds or so. Relax and enjoy the effects of your meditation.

SEVEN-WAVE SAT NAM MEDITATION

Sit in Easy Pose with a straight spine. Place the palms flat together at the center of the chest, thumbs lightly pressing into the center of the sternum. With closed eyes, look up slightly, focusing at the third-eye point. Inhale deeply. With the exhale, chant the mantra in the law of seven, or law of the tides (waves). *Sat* will vibrate in six waves, and *Nam* in the seventh.

The first wave of sound begins at the base of the spine. Then the sound moves through the sex organs, the navel point, the heart center, the throat center, and the third-eye point. On chanting *Nam*, let the energy and sound radiate from the seventh chakra, the crown center, at the top of the head through the aura. Then take another deep breath and repeat the process. Continue for 11 minutes. Build the meditation to 31 minutes. (See "Resources" section for companion CD.)

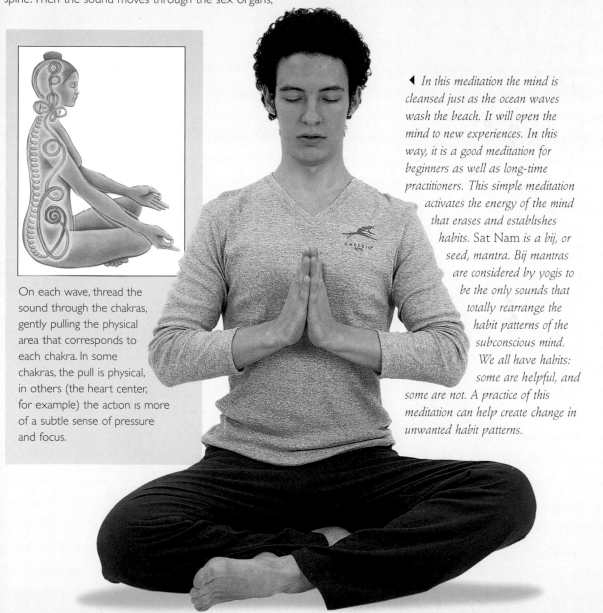

On each wave, thread the sound through the chakras, gently pulling the physical area that corresponds to each chakra. In some chakras, the pull is physical, in others (the heart center, for example) the action is more of a subtle sense of pressure and focus.

◀ *In this meditation the mind is cleansed just as the ocean waves wash the beach. It will open the mind to new experiences. In this way, it is a good meditation for beginners as well as long-time practitioners. This simple meditation activates the energy of the mind that erases and establishes habits. Sat Nam is a bij, or seed, mantra. Bij mantras are considered by yogis to be the only sounds that totally rearrange the habit patterns of the subconscious mind.*

We all have habits: some are helpful, and some are not. A practice of this meditation can help create change in unwanted habit patterns.

KIRTAN KRIYA
SA TA NA MA

This meditation employs the elementary sounds of *Sat Nam*. The power of *sa ta na ma* is likened to the energy of the atom, since the atom (or *bij*) of the sound *Sat Nam* is being broken into its nuclear parts. *Sa ta na ma* is also referred to as Kirtan Kriya, because Kirtan means "divine song," and this mantra is chanted in a simple singing style. One of Kundalini Yoga's classics, this meditation will clear the mind of subconscious "garbage," and is thus perfect to do upon rising or before going to bed. (The musical notation for this can be found on page 80, and also see Resources for companion CD.)

The a in each syllable is pronounced like *ah*. Each syllable is a sound vibration with a specific meaning. They are:

> *Sa* - the universe, totality
> *Ta* - life, creation
> *Na* - death, dissolution
> *Ma*- rebirth, regeneration

YOGA , PRESSURE POINTS, AND MERIDIANS

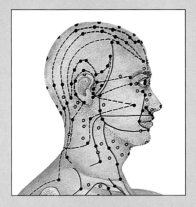

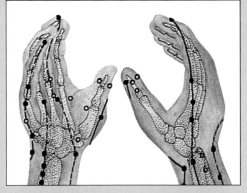

Yoga stimulates pressure points and meridians in much the same way as acupressure. When you press the fingertips in *sa ta na ma* , you activate pressure points that help the energy flow along the meridians to the brain. This activation clears the subconscious mind and alllows accesses to the higher centers of the brain.

In this meditation, you will be doing several things at once:

1 Your thumbs will sequentially press each of the fingers in the following way as you chant:

Remember that each finger reflexes to the brain, so press with enough pressure to activate the brain functions (about 5 pounds of pressure).

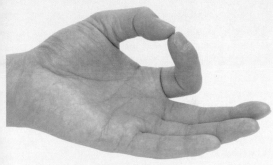

Sa - thumb and index finger (for wisdom)

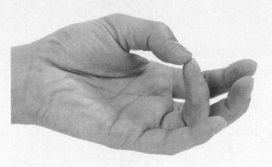

Na - thumb and ring finger (for energy)

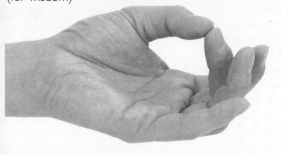

Ta - thumb and middle finger (for patience)

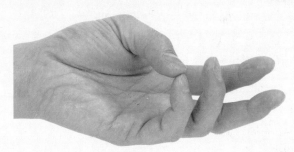

Ma - thumb and little finger (for communication)

2 There are 3 "voices" used in this meditation:

Out loud - the human voice
Whisper - the voice of the lover
Silent - the inner voice

As a beginner, chant in the out loud voice for 3 minutes, then the whisper for 3 minutes, then the silent voice for 3 minutes. Then reverse: chant in the silent voice for 3 minutes, whisper for 3, and end with chanting out loud for 3 minutes. This will total

18 minutes. You can work up to 5 minutes for each section, adding on an extra minute in the silent part, for a total of 31 minutes. Remember to continue pressing the fingers while chanting internally on the silent part.

3 Mental focus: Feel the sound of each syllable come in through the crown center, and go out through the third-eye point in an L shape. This energy flow follows the pathway called the Golden Cord, which is the connection between the pineal and the pituitary glands.

TEN STEPS TO PEACE

"This meditation takes care of phobias, fears, and neuroses. It can remove unsettling thoughts from the past that surface into the present. It can take difficult situations in the present and release them into the hands of Infinity. All this can be done in just forty seconds!"

—Yogi Bhajan

1 Sit with a straight spine in Easy Pose. Gaze at the tip of the nose with the eyes open one-tenth of the way. Mentally say Wahe Guru (Wah-hay-g'roo) in the following manner:

Wa - focus on the right eye
he - focus on the left eye
Guru - focus on the tip of the nose

Wahe Guru is the expression of ecstasy, of merger with the Infinite. In this meditation you will repeat the above process on each exhale.

2 Inhale and remember an encounter or memory that happened to you.

3 Exhale with *Wahe Guru* as before.

4 Inhale. Visualize and relive the actual feeling of the encounter.

5 Exhale with *Wahe Guru* as before.

6 Inhale and reverse roles in the encounter you are remembering. Become the other person and experience their perspective.

7 Exhale with *Wahe Guru* as before.

8 Inhale. Forgive the other person and forgive yourself.

9 Exhale with *Wahe Guru* as before.

10 Inhale. Let go of the incident and release it into the Universe.

MEDITATION TO BREAK ADDICTION

Sit in Easy Pose with a straight spine, making sure that the first six lower vertebrae are locked forward. Make fists with both hands and extend the thumbs straight. Place the thumbs on the temples, and find the niche where the thumbs fit just right.

Lock the back molars together and keep the lips closed. The molars will alternately tighten, then release; right then left, then right and so on. You should feel the alternating movement under the thumbs at the temples. Keep a firm pressure applied on the temples. Keep the mouth closed, focus at the brow point, and mentally hear the sound of *sa ta na ma*, one sound for each pressing of the molars. Continue coordinating the mantra with the subtle movement of the jaws for 5 to 7 minutes. With practice the time can be increased to 20 minutes, and ultimately to 31 minutes.

▶ *The imbalance in the pineal area upsets the pulsation of the pineal gland itself. It is this pulsation that regulates the pituitary gland, which regulates the rest of the glands. As the glands go, so follows the body and mind, thus creating an imbalance that results in unhealthy habits or addiction.*

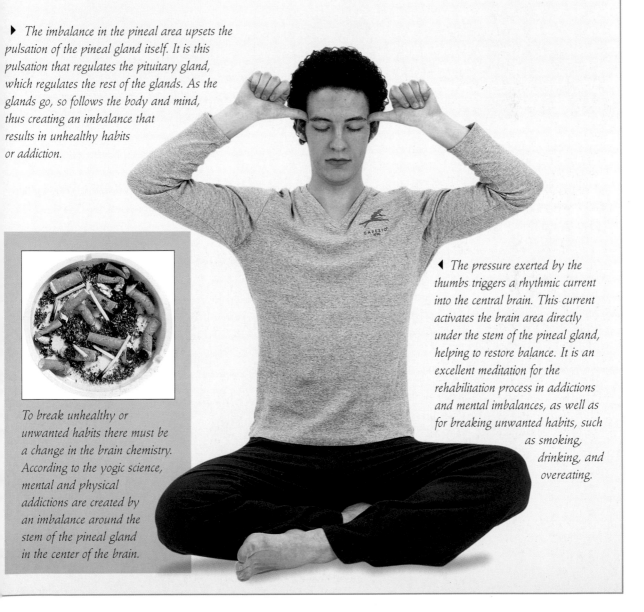

To break unhealthy or unwanted habits there must be a change in the brain chemistry. According to the yogic science, mental and physical addictions are created by an imbalance around the stem of the pineal gland in the center of the brain.

◀ *The pressure exerted by the thumbs triggers a rhythmic current into the central brain. This current activates the brain area directly under the stem of the pineal gland, helping to restore balance. It is an excellent meditation for the rehabilitation process in addictions and mental imbalances, as well as for breaking unwanted habits, such as smoking, drinking, and overeating.*

MEDITATION FOR UNWANTED THOUGHTS

Sit straight in Easy Pose. Make a cup with the hands by putting the right hand inside the left, so that when you look into this cup you see the right palm facing you. The fingers will cross each other. Put this open cup at the level of the heart center. Your eyes will only look into this cup. Keep the head straight as you gaze. Inhale deeply through the nose. Exhale through the puckered mouth into the cup. The exhalation is a long, dry spitting motion. Meditate on the particular thought that you have and do not like to have. Spit out the thought with the breath. Inhale the thought, then exhale it into the cup.

Continue for 11 minutes, then inhale deeply and exhale. With the eyes closed, begin to concentrate on the spine. Slowly draw your concentration down the spine all the way to the bottom. Feel the last vertebrae. Feel the spine as if you are feeling a stick in your hand. The more you can feel the entire spine to the base, the more the energy flow will activate your meditation.

▶ *The ancient technology of this kriya works to change a particular area of the brain where conflict in the personality sits. This area is located one-third of the way up from the base of the skull. This meditation and the following one both use the same technology, but the mental focus is different for each. They are two entirely separate meditations, and are not meant to be practiced together.*

"BEGGAR'S" MEDITATION FOR DESIRE

Sit exactly as in the Meditation for Unwanted Thoughts. Inhale deeply and exhale through the puckered mouth, a long, dry spit. Meditate on inhaling a particular desire and spit it into the cup with the breath through the mouth. Pick a single strong desire, and focus only on that desire throughout the meditation. The desire will feel calmed and fulfilled. Continue for 11 minutes, then inhale, exhale, and relax.

◀ *This meditation works on the pranic ener in the aura and affects the same area of the brain as the previous meditation. This meditation contains the technology to deal wi desire. It removes the block of too much desir that can prevent you from achieving your fullest potential. Please note that there are tw main differences between this meditation ana the previous one: one, the focus is on desires, not thoughts; and two, this meditation does not hav the final concentration on the spine that ends the previous one.*

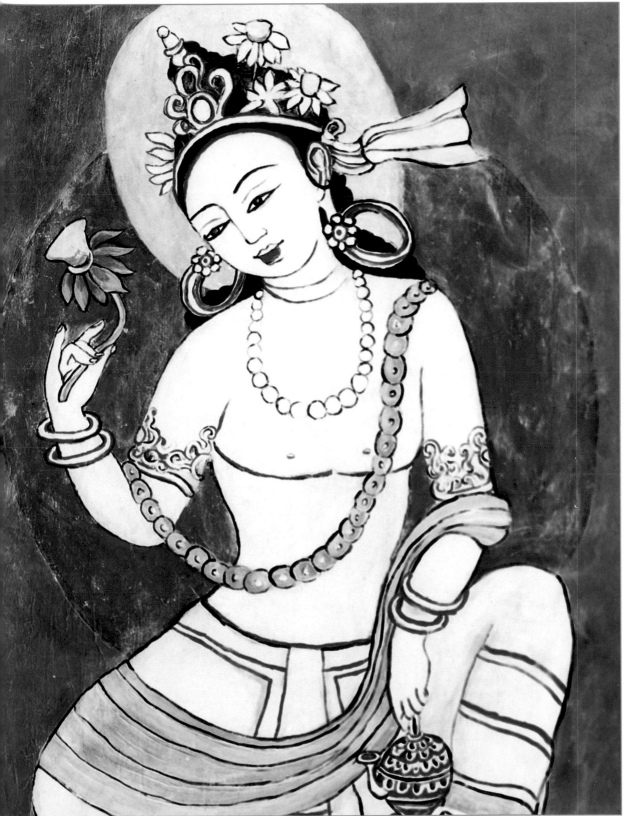

HEALING MEDITATION

Meditations with the intent to heal oneself or someone else often use the mantra of healing, *ra ma da sa, sa say so hung*. Two meditations are included here that use this mantra. (See Resources for Companion CD.) These meditations can be done in a group, with the person(s) to be healed resting in the center; or, if not physically present, resting in the visual memory of the meditators. The mantra's elementary sounds are translated as follows:

Ra - sun energy

Ma - moon energy

Da - earth energy

Sa - infinity, universal energy

Sa - repeat in second half of mantra

Say - the personal embodiment of *sa*

So - personal sense of merger with *sa*

Hung - the Infinite, vibrating and real

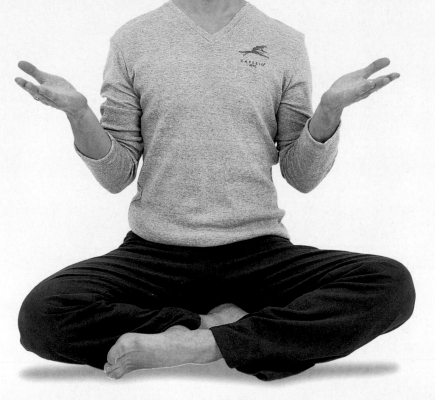

Sit in Easy Pose with a straight spine. Bend the arms and bring the elbows against the sides of the rib cage. The palms of the hands face the sky and are flat, with the wrists pressed back to a 45° angle to the sides of the body. The eyes are closed and focused at the third-eye point. Repeat the mantra once per breath in the following manner.

On the first *Sa* and on *Hung*, pull in on the navel point. These two syllables will be abbreviated, with the sound *Hung* vibrated at the root of the nose. The rest of the syllables are drawn out in a strong, powerful chant that uses all the breath for each repetition of the mantra. Continue for 5 to 11 minutes, increasing gradually up to 31 minutes. Inhale, hold the breath, and circulate the healing energy or send it to the person you are concentrating on for healing. Exhale and relax.

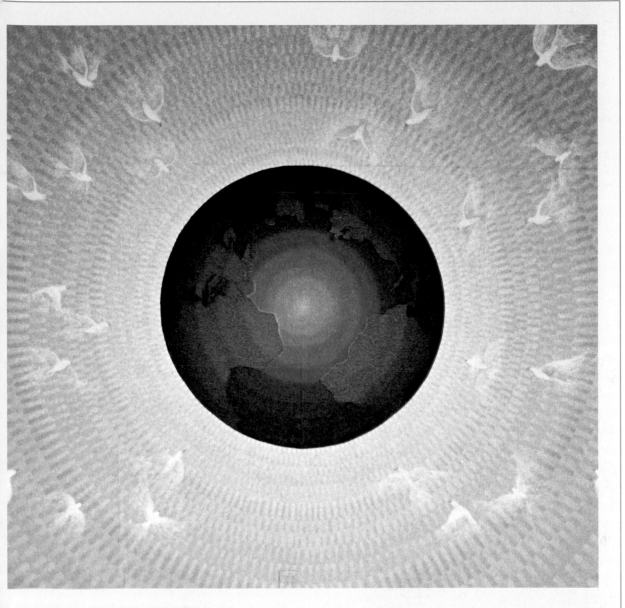

HEALING OUR PLANET

We can help our planet and all living things on it, just by
directing our good will toward it. Using meditation to send
healing energy and prayers to our planet creates an energy
field that affects the whole earth.

Use the *ra ma da sa* healing meditation given previously,
or sit meditatively and simply affrirm "God bless this earth
with peace," or "May peace prevail on Earth." Repeat
one round of the mantra or affirmation per breath for
11 minutes or more. Sit in a circle and visualize the earth
in the center for a powerful group meditation.

Sat Nam Rasayan (Rah sah-yan) literally, "universal
remedy of manifested truth," is the healing branch
of Kundalini Yoga, dating back to the sixteenth-
century Indian saint and Sikh master, Guru Ram
Das. In this meditative approach, the healer opens
to a sensitive process of awareness, creating a
sacred space in which healing can occur naturally.
(See "Resources" for books and training programs.)

On exhaling, the air is pushed out from the lungs as the diaphragm moves upward.

RESPIRATION AND SUSPENSION OF BREATH

Briefly suspending the breath on either the inhalation or exhalation pauses the breathing process, and allows the oxygen to circulate deeply throughout the body and mind.

◀ *The yogic teachings say that if you slow the breath down to 1 per minute, you will experience the meditative mind, be calm and happy, and never be short of energy. Prana (life force) and apana (eliminated energy) are used efficiently in this exercise, as you take a deep, slow breath in, hold it and circulate the prana, exhale deeply and slowly, and hold out, circulating the apana.*

ONE MINUTE BREATH

Sit in Easy Pose with a straight spine. Place the hands in Gian Mudra with the arms relaxed but straight. You may need to keep your eyes slightly open if using a timer to monitor your breath, or you can count silently (one way to count seconds is to mentally repeat "one thousand one, one thousand two," etc.) Inhale deeply and slowly, using the yogic abdominal breathing. As you suspend the inhalation, bring your attention to the upper ribs and clavicle. Lift the upper ribs slightly and fix them in place. Relax the shoulders and face. Allow the belly to relax slightly outward. Finally, pull the chin in slightly. Become still and calm. Exhale slowly. Press the remaining breath out in small stages to empty completely. Suspend the breath out. Relax your shoulders, face, and upper chest. The abdominal muscles will be pressed in slightly and relaxed.

Your brain will trigger you to breathe when the level of carbon dioxide in the blood rises. If you prepare to suspend the breath by taking several exhalations (blowing out the carbon dioxide), you will hold the breath longer and with more comfort. With the breath suspended in, when you at first feel like exhaling, inhale a little bit more to remain in the suspended breath mode a little longer. This can extend the length of the suspension without any strain.

Ideally, the breath is inhaled for 20 seconds, held in the body for 20 seconds, exhaled for 20 seconds, totaling 1 minute. Beginners should cut each section to 8 to 10 seconds for each part and increase slowly and gradually by adding a few seconds to each part over time. Under no circumstances should you hold the breath to the point of dizziness or faintness.

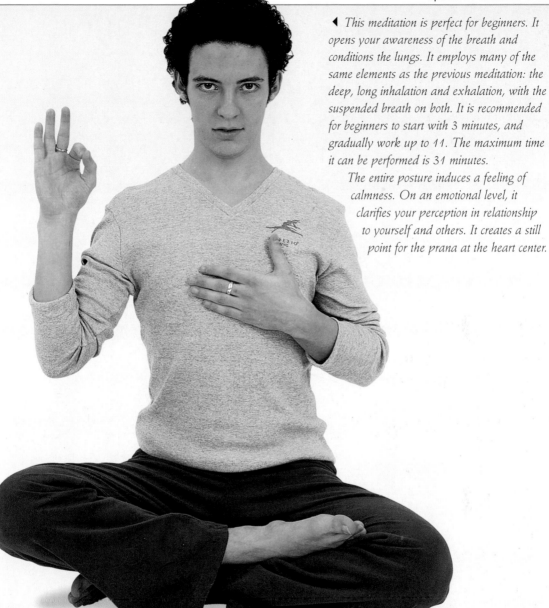

◀ *This meditation is perfect for beginners. It opens your awareness of the breath and conditions the lungs. It employs many of the same elements as the previous meditation: the deep, long inhalation and exhalation, with the suspended breath on both. It is recommended for beginners to start with 3 minutes, and gradually work up to 11. The maximum time it can be performed is 31 minutes.*

The entire posture induces a feeling of calmness. On an emotional level, it clarifies your perception in relationship to yourself and others. It creates a still point for the prana at the heart center.

FOR A CALM HEART

Sit in Easy Pose with the spine straight. Either close the eyes or look straight ahead with the eyes half open. Place the left hand on the center of the chest at the heart-center level. The palm is flat against the chest and the fingers are parallel to the ground, pointing to the right. The right hand is raised up to the right side of the body as if taking an oath. The palm is facing forward, and the first finger is curled into the thumb in active Gian Mudra. The rest of the fingers are straight. The forearm is perpendicular to the ground. Concentrate on the flow of the breath. Feel it consciously. Inhale slowly and deeply through the nose. Suspend the breath as it is locked in. Retain the breath as long as possible. Then exhale smoothly, gradually, and completely. When the breath is totally exhaled, suspend the breath out for as long as possible. Continue this pattern for a specified amount of time, then inhale, exhale strongly 3 times, and relax.

MEDITATION TO MAKE THE IMPOSSIBLE POSSIBLE (GAN PATTEE)

This meditation has three parts. The first part uses the *sa ta na ma* mantra, combined with the *ra ma da sa, sa say so hung* mantra. This combines the subconscious cleansing properties of *sa ta na ma*, with the self-healing properties of the *ra na da sa* meditation. In Gan Pattee, you "sing" the mantra in the same style as in *sa ta na ma*, and touch each finger to the thumb as you chant, as in *sa ta na ma*. For each repetition of the mantra, the fingers will be pressed in three rounds: *sa ta na ma* equals 1 round, *ra ma da sa* equals 2 rounds, and *sa say so hung* is the 3rd round.

▼ *When you don't know what to do and nothing is working right,* Gan Pattee Kriya *(pronounced gun put-tee) will bring you victory. It will take away past and present negativity, smooth out your day-to-day problems, and help you create a positive tomorrow.*

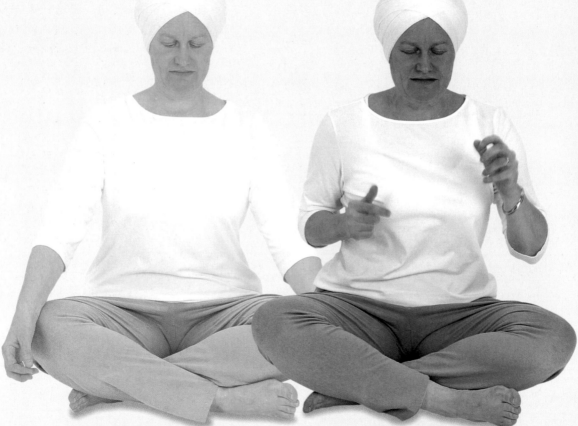

Sit with a straight spine. Bring the hands to the knees with the fingers outstretched and the arms straight. The eyes are one-tenth open and gazing at the top of the nose. Begin to press the fingers as you chant the mantra, 1 repetition on each breath. Take a deep breath in between each repetition. Continue for 11 minutes, and slowly work up to 31 minutes of practice.

At the end of 11 minutes, stay sitting and inhale deeply. Hold the breath for 20 to 30 seconds while you move every part of your body. Shake, jump, and wiggle every inch of yourself, then exhale. Inhale and repeat the process 2 more times to circulate the prana to every part of the body. This is for self-healing.

Sit totally still in absolute calmness. Concentrate on the tip of your nose with the eyes one-tenth open for 1 minute. (See Resources for companion CD.)

RHYTHMIC BREATH MEDITATION (SHABD KRIYA)

Sit in a comfortable position with the spine straight. Place the hands in the lap, palms upward, with the right hand over the left, so that when you look down at the hands you will be looking at the right palm. The thumbs are together and straight, pointing slightly away from you. Gaze at the tip of the nose, the eyelids half-closed.

Inhale in 4 equal parts, mentally hearing the sound *sa ta na ma*. Hold the breath, mentally repeating the mantra 4 times for a total of 16 beats. Then exhale in 2 equal strokes projecting mentally *Wahe Guru* (Wa-hey the first stroke, G'roo the second). Continue for 11 minutes. Slowly and gradually work up to 31 minutes.

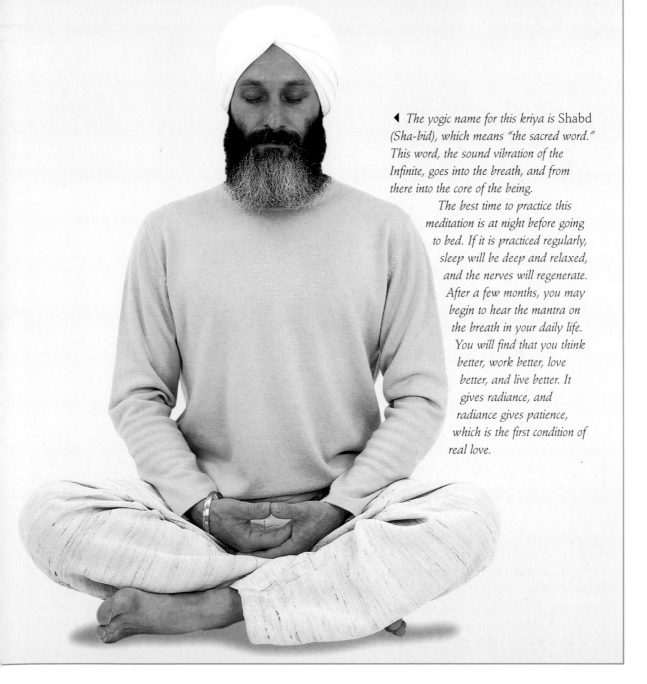

◀ *The yogic name for this kriya is Shabd (Sha-bid), which means "the sacred word." This word, the sound vibration of the Infinite, goes into the breath, and from there into the core of the being.*

The best time to practice this meditation is at night before going to bed. If it is practiced regularly, sleep will be deep and relaxed, and the nerves will regenerate. After a few months, you may begin to hear the mantra on the breath in your daily life. You will find that you think better, work better, love better, and live better. It gives radiance, and radiance gives patience, which is the first condition of real love.

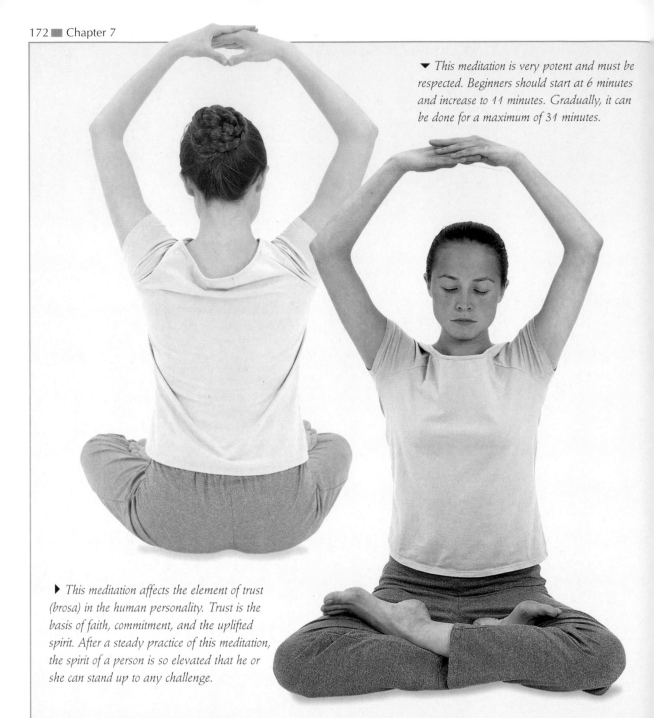

▼ *This meditation is very potent and must be respected. Beginners should start at 6 minutes and increase to 11 minutes. Gradually, it can be done for a maximum of 31 minutes.*

▶ *This meditation affects the element of trust (brosa) in the human personality. Trust is the basis of faith, commitment, and the uplifted spirit. After a steady practice of this meditation, the spirit of a person is so elevated that he or she can stand up to any challenge.*

MEDITATION FOR TRUST

Sit in Lotus or Easy Pose. Arch the arms up over the head with the palms down. Men will put the right palm on top of the left. Women will put the left palm on top of the right. Put the thumb tips together with the thumbs pointing back. The arms are bent slightly, and the hands are 6-8 inches above the head. Keep a pressure on the arms to maintain the arch. The eyes are open slightly and look down toward the upper lip. Begin to whisper the mantra *Wahe Guru* (Wah hey G'roo). Form the sounds with the lips and tongue very precisely. Whisper so that *Guru* is almost inaudible. Continue at a rate of about 2½ seconds per repetition.

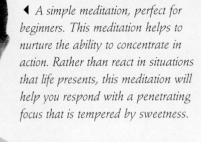

◀ *A simple meditation, perfect for beginners. This meditation helps to nurture the ability to concentrate in action. Rather than react in situations that life presents, this meditation will help you respond with a penetrating focus that is tempered by sweetness.*

FOR FOCUS AND SWEETNESS

Sit comfortably in Easy Pose, with a straight spine. With the four fingers of the right hand, feel the pulse on the left wrist. Once you find the position of the strongest pulse, place the fingers in a straight line, pressing lightly so that you can feel the pulse in each fingertip. With each beat of the pulse, mentally hear *Sat Nam*. Close the eyes, and gently focus at the third-eye point, where the eyebrows meet the nose. Continue for 11 minutes, gradually increasing the time up to 31 minutes.

THE MORNING CALL (LONG EK ONG KAR MEDITATION)

This meditation is considered a classic in Kundalini Yoga. It was one of the first meditations taught by Yogi Bhajan. The best time to practice this meditation is in the early hours of the morning, called the *Amrit Vela* (the ambrosial hours), before sunrise. In the quiet of that special time of the day, the earth's vibratory energy is poised for all the possibilities of that day. For this reason, this meditation is often referred to as The Morning Call.

Long Ek Ong Kar opens the chakras and energizes your higher awareness. The extended sounds allow for a deep meditation. *Ek Ong Kar* means "One Creator/Creation." *Sat Nam* means "Truth-Identity," and *Siri Wahe Guru* means "Great beyond description is Divine Wisdom."

Sit with a straight spine. Bring the hands into Gian Mudra and close the eyes. Inhale deeply and chant *Ek* from the navel center, then smoothly move into *Ong,* leaving just enough breath to chant *Kar* for about the same length of time as *Ong.* Take another deep breath and chant *Sat* from the navel, then resound *Nam* in a long tone resounding from the heart center. At the end, when there is little breath left, chant *Siri* (pronounced with a rolled *r*). Then take a half-breath and chant *Wha* (a short sound, somewhat aspirated), then *Hay* (also short), followed by *G'roo*, which extends slightly. Inhale deeply and repeat the cycle. Continue for 11 minutes. (See "Resources" for companion CD.)

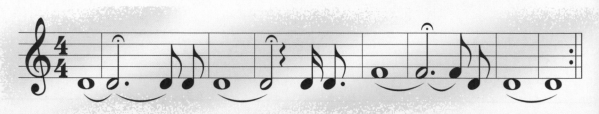

ong...   namo...   guroo dev...   namo...

Ram Das means "one who serves God," and can refer to a Sikh master known for his humility, service, and healing qualities.

SINGING FROM THE HEART

Many meditations included in this book have mantras that are chanted in a monotone. Another approach to meditation is to sing. Singing meditations open the heart as well as the lungs. Singing activates our eighth body, the pranic body, which brings fearless living. Singing songs of simple goodness and truth channel our emotions into a devotion to the highest, in ourselves and others.

One of the most commonnly sung mantras is *Guru Guru Wahe Guru, Guru Ram Das Guru* (G'roo G'roo Wa Hay G'roo, G'roo Raam Daas G'roo). The first part of the mantra affirms the infinite, absolute Creator. The second part recognizes the personal relationship we have with the Creator within and without. Many stories have been told of miraculous healing and transformation by people who have changed this mantra in sincerity and devotion. This mantra calls forth the power of healing energy and protection from negativity. (See "Resources" for companion CD.)

VISUALIZATIONS

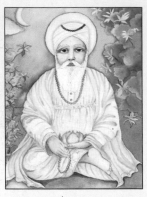

To visualize is to imagine, to evoke, to conceive. Visualizing as a form of meditation uses the imagination to evoke changes within the psyche, to conceive and give birth to a new state of consciousness. Visualizing as meditation involves more than the internal sense of seeing. In order to truly visualize, you need to feel. Scenes can unfold in your mind's "eye," yet without involving yourself through your feelings, it is hardly more than watching a television screen. To make it real, you must feel. Use all of your senses—touch, smell, hear, and feel your way through your experience.

During visualization, you can either sit in a meditative pose with the spine straight, or lie down in Corpse Pose on the back. Upon completing the visualization, if in Corpse Pose, do the wake-up exercises. If you are sitting up, take some deep breaths and stretch your body up, shaking your arms and hands.

In order to keep a meditative state while visualizing, it is suggested that you have someone slowly read the visualization out loud, or play a recording of it. The very best for self-healing is to listen to a playback of your own voice guiding you through these visualizations.

The first two visualizations are given in Yogi Bhajan's own words. The third is a journey to a place of healing.

Visualization on the Heart Lotus

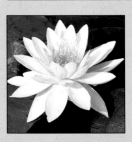

"Meditate for peace, tranquility, happiness, joy, and bliss. Feel the energy of the sun and moon, the universe, all planets, all gods and goddesses, saints and sages, all good people, all kind people, all grateful people. They are all radiating the energy to you, and you are receiving peace. Fill yourself and take a part out of the universe and its nectar. Just meditate, and the petals of the flowers are being showered on you throughout the heavens by all the saints and sages, holy men, gods and goddesses. People of dignity and grace and virtue are showering blessings on you. We are blessed by Guru and gurus, and by all those who came throughout time and gave the message of God. They are all radiating their light to you, and you are vibrating under that radiation.

"Meditate and feel that the lotus of the heart is turning upwards, the fragrance is spreading all around you, and that you can smell a special smell of you, a fragrance of you. Feel the kindness of those great ones who attuned their lives to righteousness. Feel that they are in you, are around you, are by your side, and that radiance of their auras is filling up your mind.

"Focus your eyes at the tip of your nose and feel that the power of the universe is coming into you. Now radiate, and feel that all that radiance is making your life in this body transparent, and all opaqueness is vanishing. You are becoming transparent. Inhale deep . . . exhale. Inhale deep . . . exhale. Inhale deep . . . exhale."

—Yogi Bhajan

You Are the Universe

Sit down and close your eyes. Utilize your energy. All minds can do it. That is a guaranteed fact. Sit down in a posture that is convenient to your body, your spine as straight as you can possibly make it. That is the first requirement, that your posture should be graceful, steady, and convenient. Second is, close your eyes and go within. Your eyes must open your inner eye. Outer eyes must not see.

"Now start imagining that you are the greatest self-enlightened being. You are great, great, great, great, whatever it is . . . a perfectly enlightened being. Your body can be stilled at your command. Your nerves are under your supervision. Your thoughts are under your control. You are mentally, physically, and spiritually a being that knows all about everything. You shall not limit your thinking about greatness. Flood yourself with the thought that you are the greatest. You are the universe, you are the Infinite One. You are the Being of the beings, the Supreme Being. Take your mind to that thought.

"I know, a lot of problems will happen on the way if you try to think that way. First, the ego will say, 'Hey man, you have been worshiping so and so all your life, now you say you are greater than that? What nonsense is this?' A lot of negative thoughts will cross your mind, but you'll cross all of them. Keep on growing. Whosoever put you here, put you here for growth. All He wanted was for you to be here to find a place. The growth is always His, and He will take care of your mental growth and your levitated form as a being.

"Delicately transfer yourself. Expand yourself. Pull yourself systematically: 'I made this planet, I made these mountains with snow peaks, I made this forest, ocean, people, animal kingdom.' Think, as God, what you have done, who you are, what you are. Nobody can question you. You are Omnipresent, Omniscient, Omnicompetent. You can never realize about somebody's greatness if you have never had to work yourself into that position. Just meditate and realize yourself as God through all the beauty and magnificence and the totality of this universe. Concentrate and think, and imagine, and grow . . ."

—Yogi Bhajan

THE HEALING WATERS OF THE GOLDEN TEMPLE

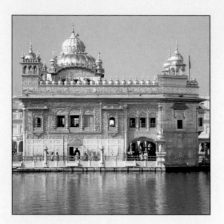

Golden Temple

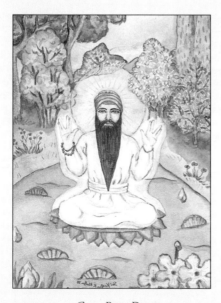

Guru Ram Das

In the Punjab of Northern India, a sparkling jewel-like temple sits healing water called the Tank of Nectar by those who know it. It said that thousands of years ago, this very same water brought Lc Rama's sons to life when sprinkled on them. Others say that Lord Buddha visited the pool and claimed it to be a blessed place to attain enlightenment.

In the 16th century, a miracle occurred in which a leper was cured by dipping in this water. The fourth of the Sikh masters, Gu Ram Das, recognized this miracle as the sign he had anticipated t begin to build a temple of gold with a healing tank of water surrounding it. In 1573 the spot was excavated and Amritsar, the Tank of Nectar, was born. The Golden Temple, a delicately beautif temple inlaid with gold, sits as a golden heart nested in the cente of the water. The Golden Temple was built with four open doors, one on each side, to signify that the temple would always be ope to all paths. Almost 24 hours a day, there is beautiful music, called kirtan; sacred songs float out and over the healing water, touching the souls of all who walk the marble walkway around the pool o water.

In our meditative journey we will visualize going inside the Golden Temple to meditate, then walking outside to dip in the healing water. When you visualize, know that although your physic body remains either lying or sitting on the ground, your other bodies—the mental, the spiritual, the subtle—are taking you where you will them to go. Trust that you are experiencing the reality of the journey, and you will.

Lie down on your back or sit in a meditative posture, with the body or spine covered with a light shawl. If possible, have music playing softly, especially the "Guru Ram Das Chant" or a sacred song of the Sikhs, to set the atmosphere. (See "Resources" for companion CD.)

Begin to let your body sink into the ground, Allow your mind to do the same. Breathe gently — long and light breaths that carry your spirit to the Golden Temple. Feel the air on your skin. Take in the smells of India, smells of the dusty earth mixed with a sweetness that recalls flowers and honey. Hear the music as if in the distance. Feel the call of the heart to go toward it. Walk with freshly washed bare feet on the cool marble that covers the entire walkway around the tank of water. See the shimmering reflection of the Golden Temple dance on the water. Your ears are filled with the sounds of sacred music, at once expressing both the human longing to merge with the Infinite and the ecstatic experience of that merger. Walk the narrow walkway up to the entrance, and go through the doorway into the golden inner room. Sit and meditate in the uplifted energy of the place, along with so many others who are answering the call of their soul. Stay in the golden light as long as you like.

When you are ready, move to the marble walkway, cool and smooth to the foot's touch. Walk to where you can rest under the very same tree that was there when the tank was discovered. Walk down the stairs into the cool, silky water. Feel it all around you, and feel it inside of you. Dip down and give your need, your longing, to the water. Think of those whom you want to bless, and dip in the water for them. Dip for the whole earth, if you wish to. Experience yourself letting go, surrendering into the cool healing water. Stay as long as you like. Then come out slowly, and wrap yourself in a shawl. See yourself sitting or lying down in the warm sun. Feel the warmth of the sun shining in your heart and radiating out to everyone. Feel your gratitude for your life, and send a blessing to all.

Stay as long as you like, and when you are ready, feel yourself slowly and gently come back to the place where your body is resting, or sitting. Breathe consciously and deeply and begin the wake-up exercises. Take your time, and keep the essence of your experience with you as you go through your day.

CHAPTER 8

THE YOGA OF DAILY LIFE

"Life is like a nest which must be
built straw by straw."

–Yogi Bhajan

RISE AND SHINE
IN THE MORNING

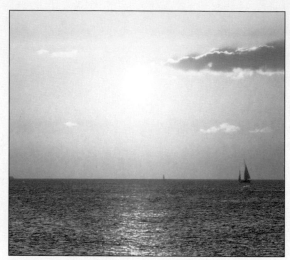

Yoga is a way of life. Beside the well-known element of yoga postures, there are yogic teachings for virtually every aspect of human existence. There is a yogic way to get up in the morning, to go to bed at night, and to take care of the body. The yogic science provides effective, efficient, and enlightened ways of conducting everyday life. Based on each individual's inclination, the following yogic teachings can be incorporated into daily life.

According to the ancient teachings, a very special time of the day occurs when the sun is at a 60° angle to the earth. This happens twice a day: before sunrise and at sunset. The angle created by the sun at those times has different energetic qualities. At predawn, between the hours of 4 and 6 A.M., the earth is quiet and the magnetic energy is influenced by the sun's angle in somewhat the same way the earth's tides are affected by the moon. This is the best time to meditate, to practice yoga, and to clear the subconscious mind. The Sanskrit name for this practice is **Sadhana** (Saad-na), and it means daily spiritual practice—particularly in the early morning hours.

Many times you may have wakened at that time of the day and noticed that you had just been in a highly active dream state. Upon a closer look, you may have found that your dreams were playing out subconscious thoughts. If, instead of sleeping and remaining in an unconscious state of mind, you were to rise and meditate, those subconscious thoughts would present themselves to your conscious mind. Through meditation, they can be released, and the subconscious mind cleansed.

Ideally your yoga and meditation practice is done before dawn for the most powerful effects. But no matter what time it is done, establishing a practice in the morning before starting the day will greatly benefit the quality of your life. Following are some helpful yogic tips on how to get started in the morning.

1 **When** you get a mental signal to wake up, keep your eyes closed and stretch your hands over your head to channel the magnetic energy of the earth. Then cup your hands and place them over your eyes. Open your eyes slowly and look into your cupped hands. This allows your eyes to focus gently, and to adjust to any light in the room. Then place your hands on your eyes and gently massage the rest of your face.

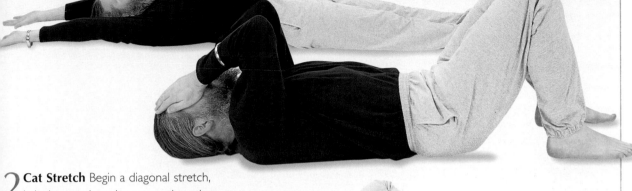

2 **Cat Stretch** Begin a diagonal stretch, bringing one bent leg across the other. Twist to the side. Repeat on the other side. This stretches and wakes up the spine.

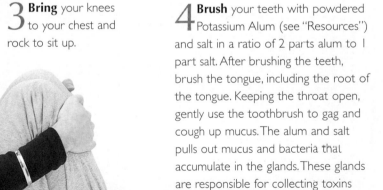

3 **Bring** your knees to your chest and rock to sit up.

4 **Brush** your teeth with powdered Potassium Alum (see "Resources") and salt in a ratio of 2 parts alum to 1 part salt. After brushing the teeth, brush the tongue, including the root of the tongue. Keeping the throat open, gently use the toothbrush to gag and cough up mucus. The alum and salt pulls out mucus and bacteria that accumulate in the glands. These glands are responsible for collecting toxins that have drained overnight. The eyes will water, which will clean them and help to prevent cataracts.

5 **Drink** at least one glass of spring water to neutralize and ground yourself.

6 **According** to the yogic understanding of the human body, hair is the antennae of pranic energy, so it is valued and kept. Uncut hair collects pure protein at its root, which supports the brain. The hair on the head is combed with a wooden comb, to neutralize static electricity, and coiled on the highest chakra, the crown center. This takes the "antennae" and unifies them at the highest center, bringing energy to the master gland, the pineal. To protect the antennae and stabilize the brain, neurological system, and electromagnetic field, the yogic science instructs one to cover the head with a cotton cloth. The wrapped headdress automatically gives a cranial self-adjustment. The energy then becomes focused, giving one the power of penetrating projection.

Hair grows on almost all places on the human body, and in the science of yoga, it serves the purpose of drawing energy into each area, and protecting it. By keeping the body as natural as possible, we benefit from the good health that goes along with our understanding of the perfection of our natural selves.

7 **The science** of hydrotherapy has been known since ancient times. Warm showers can be used at other times of the day, but in the morning a brief, cold shower is best. Cold water opens the capillaries and strengthens the entire nervous system. When you take a cold shower, your blood rushes out to meet the challenge. This means that all the capillaries open up and all deposits and toxins are cleansed out. When the capillaries return to normal, the blood supply goes back to the organs. Each organ has its own blood supply. The cold shower thus helps flush the organs clean, like a beautiful rain helps grow the fertile crops. When the organs are flushed, the glands immediately have to change their secretion. The glands are the guardians of health, and when they change, youth returns. According to the science of yoga, youth is measured by how vibrant and healthy the glandular system is.

When you are under a cold shower, your body will feel the cold. But if given enough time, the blood and capillaries will open to the maximum and the body will not feel cold. If you bring your body to that temperature, where it can meet the cold by its own circulatory power, you have won the day. You have empowered your own health and happiness.

USING HYDROTHERAPY

Note: Pregnant and menstruating women should take warm showers.

Oil

First massage your body with pure oil; almond is preferred for its high mineral content. The oil will be driven into the skin through the pores while showering, and it will provide a protective coating to the skin.

Shower Shorts

Using a pair of mid-thigh or knee length underwear or shorts while in the shower will protect the femur bone in the thigh, which controls the calcium-magnesium balance in the body. If none are available, try to keep the thighs out of the direct spray of the water.

Shower

Allow the cold water to hit your feet, both bottoms and tops, and then the rest of your body, including your face (but not your whole head). Massage youself as you move in and out from the cold water. Pay special attention to the lymph nodes under the armpits to help prevent colds. Women should massage the breasts under the cold water to keep circulation strong. Yogis also believe this can help keep cancer away. Breathe deeply or chant a mantra to keep yourself going. Start at 30 seconds, and work up to 1 to 2 minutes. Towel dry, rubbing the skin briskly.

Dress in breathable, preferably cotton, clothing. Then you are ready for Sadhana, and ready for your day.

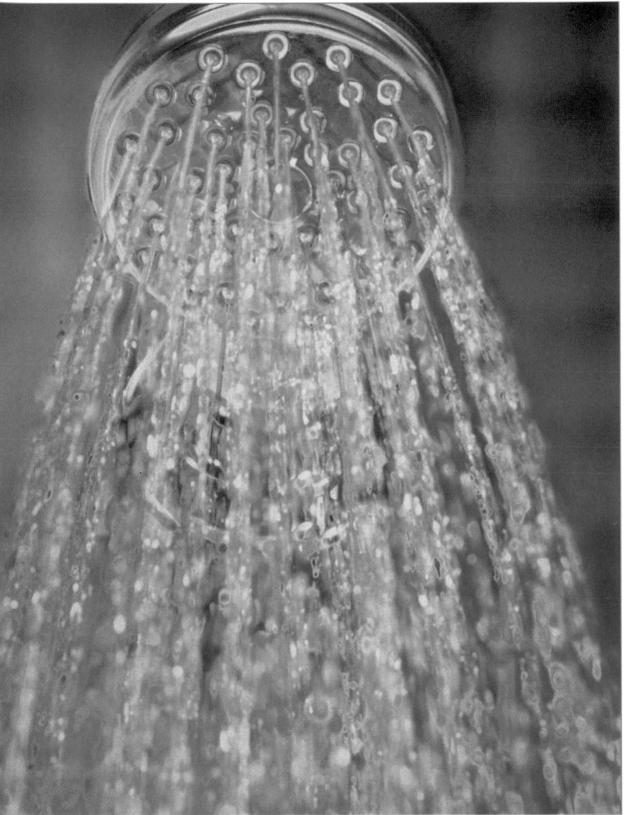

STAYING RELAXED
THROUGHOUT
THE DAY

The real tests in life come when we are faced with challenges in our workplace, our homes, or in the many roles we play throughout the day. Here are some ways the essence of yoga can keep you relaxed and uplifted.

IN THE CAR:

• Take a deep breath before driving. Say a prayer or affirmation of protection as you turn the key in the ignition.

• While sitting at a stoplight or in unmoving traffic, relax your eyes by doing the following movements with the eyes: look up, blink, look to the side, blink, look down, blink, look to the other side, blink. Then reverse the direction. This exercises and relaxes your eyes.

• Take your tongue and roll it over the outside of your teeth in a large circle. Keep the mouth closed and stretch the tongue. Go a few times, then reverse the direction. This relaxes your jaws and lower face. You may feel like yawning. A yawn should never be stifled. It is your body's way of gaining oxygen and relaxing.

• Hum along with relaxing music. Humming is soothing to the nerves, which is why people instinctively hum while rocking babies to sleep. If you need to let out tension, sing along with your favorite music as loud as you want. Chanting and singing elevated music will release tension and open the heart at the same time.

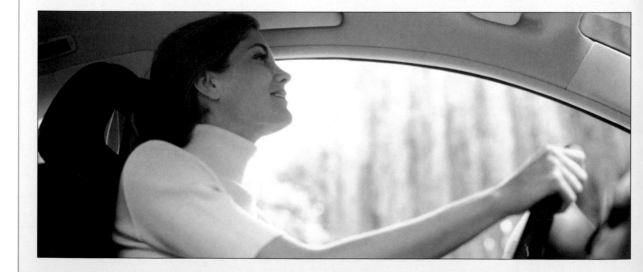

AT THE OFFICE:

• Type with the pads of the fingers, not the tips, to protect the sensitive tips and the brain areas they reflex to.

• Get up every few hours and stretch down to your feet. Breathe deeply and hang forward or hold onto the desk and stretch. Roll your head around on your neck slowly in both directions.

•Anytime during the day that your feel tired or depressed, drink a full glass of water. After working for a few hours on the computer, take a break and put a cold, wet paper towel on your face, eyes, and back of neck, and wash your hands in cold water. This is to protect your nervous system from the effects of the magnetic field of the computer.

•At least once a day, move 8 feet or more away from the computer and eat fruit for rejuvenation.

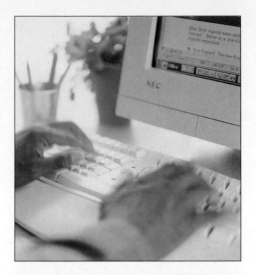

WHILE WALKING:

• Choose a mantra and walk while chanting. *Wa-hey Guru* or *Har, Haray, Haree, Wa-hey Guru* fit very well with a lively step. Chant with the beat of your step, then inhale for 4 counts and begin again. You can chant out loud, under your breath, or silently. (See "Resource" section for Breathwalk training.)

• Go out in nature and have a conversation with yourself and your creator.

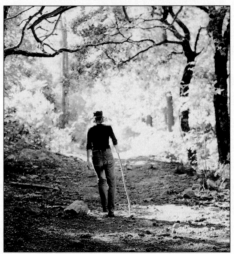

AT HOME:

• Keep elevated music playing softly throughout the day and night. (See "Resource" section for companion CD.)

• Recognize when you are beginning to feel out of balance emotionally and mentally. Excuse yourself for a few minutes, drink some water, and go to a private place. Sit and breathe long and deep, or do Breath of Fire. Talk to yourself as your own best friend.

• Eat a few raisins in the late afternoon for energy.

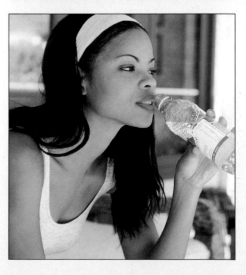

SLEEP
IN PEACE

Many people never truly relax, even when they sleep. This bedtime routine will enable you to fully relax and enter deep sleep at your will.

• Eat your final meal 3 to 4 hours before going to bed. If you eat early, your digestive system will be free to rest during the night.

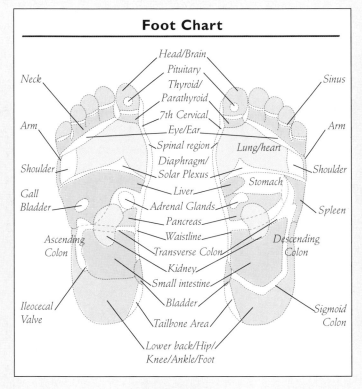

Foot Chart

Head/Brain
Pituitary
Neck
Thyroid/
Parathyroid
Sinus
7th Cervical
Arm
Eye/Ear
Arm
Spinal region
Diaphragm/
Lung/heart
Shoulder
Solar Plexus
Shoulder
Stomach
Gall
Liver
Bladder
Adrenal Glands
Spleen
Pancreas
Ascending
Waistline
Descending
Colon
Transverse Colon
Colon
Kidney
Ileocecal
Small intestine
Valve
Bladder
Sigmoid
Tailbone Area
Colon
Lower back/Hip/
Knee/Ankle/Foot

• Wash your feet with cold water in the warm weather, and warm water in the cold weather. Massage them as you wash.

• Giving and getting a full foot massage is an excellent way to end the evening. All 72,000 nerve endings are in the feet, and they all reflex to every part of the body. Relaxation of the entire nervous system is possible with proper foot massage

• Comb your hair with a wooden comb, and braid it if long enough. This consolidates the "antennae," and keeps the hair from tangling and breaking.

• Have some soothing, spiritual music playing softly through the night.

• Drink a glass of cool water before bed.

•Have your bed aligned with the electromagnetic energy poles of the earth by positioning it east-west rather than north-south. This will help you to have a deep, restful sleep and to rise easily in the morning.

•Lie down on the bed on the stomach first, with the head turned to one side to relax the body and allow it to sink into the bed. When almost asleep, turn onto your right side so that the left nostril will be dominant, providing the relaxation needed for deep sleep. Sleep with the intention of rising early to do your yoga practice.

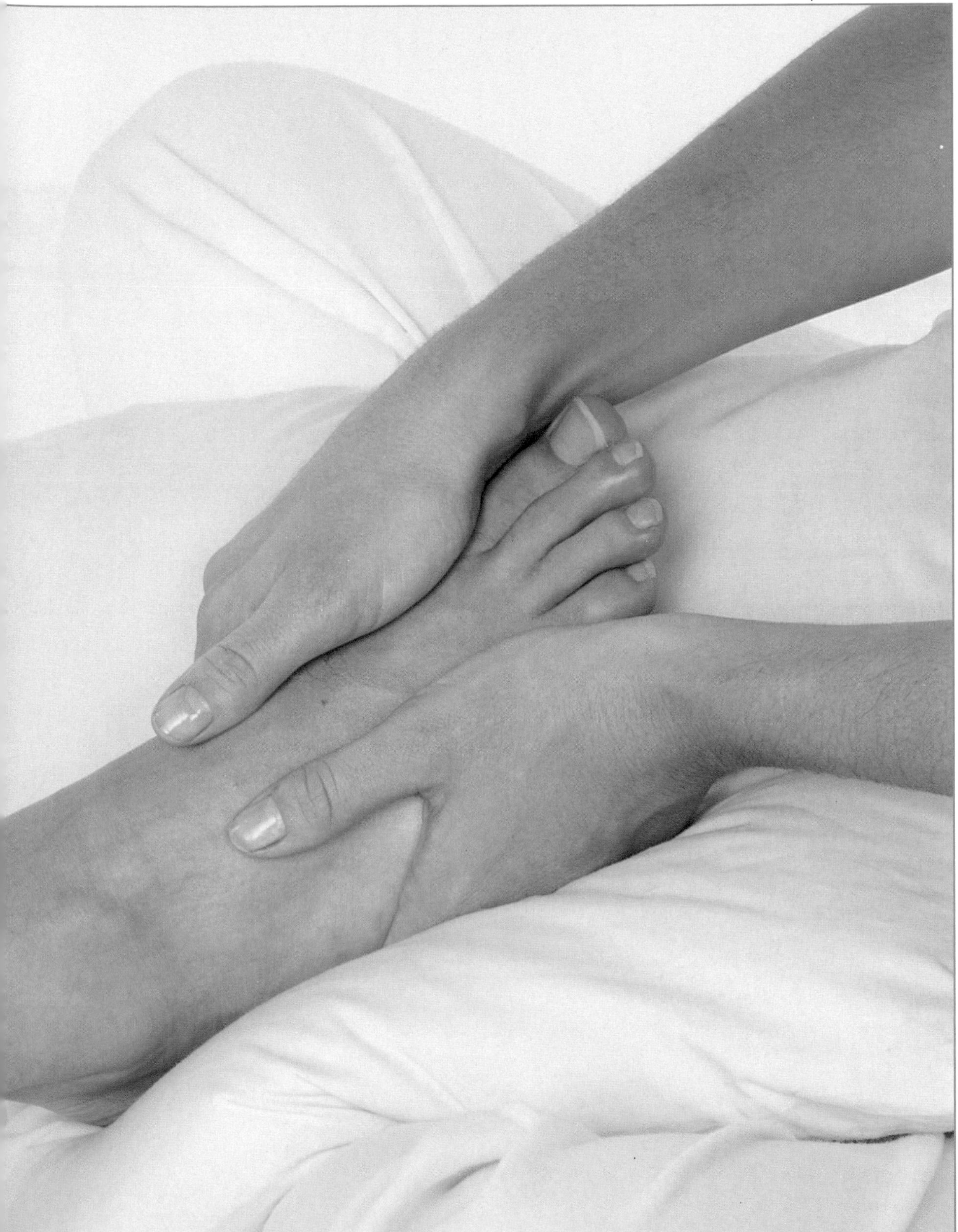

YOGA FOR
COUPLES

From the yogic perspective, a marriage is a carriage toward Infinity. It is the yoga of all yogas. As partners, we mirror each other's best and worst qualities. Marriage offers the opportunity to transform the worst to the best. Toward this end, a steady yoga practice will be invaluable.

To unite as one spirit in two bodies creates a potent and wholly satisfying energy that goes beyond what one individual is able to manifest. In marriage, challenges will always arise, but if it is the couple's intention to heal, grow, and enjoy the process, the following meditations will serve that end.

These kriyas are to be practiced with the intention to blend polarity energies for spiritual growth. Begin by using the Tuning In process (page 44). Then choose from this sampling of kriyas for couples. Since they are individual exercises and not a set, it is not necessary to do all of them together. Let your higher awareness guide you to the one(s) that will deliver the desired outcome.

LOOK INTO THE HEART

1 Lotus Flower: Sit in Easy Pose or Lotus Pose across from your partner. Sit so that your knees are almost touching. Adjust your height using a pillow if you cannot comfortably see into each other's eyes. Form your hands into a lotus flower by putting the base of the hands and wrists together, then spreading the hands open to form a cup. The little fingers will be close together. The man puts his little fingers under the woman's. These are the only fingers that touch, creating a heart lotus. Look into the heart, the soul, of your partner through the eyes. Continue for 1½ minutes.

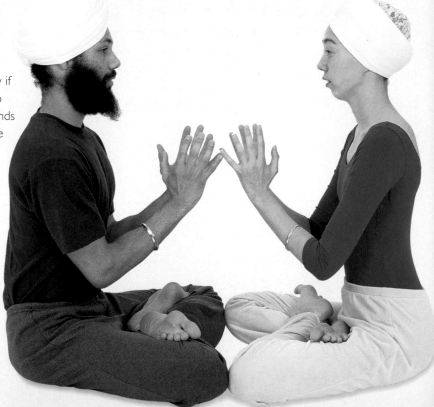

▼ This kriya slows you down from your busy daily lives, and brings an awareness of the shared heart.

There is no way you can understand the impact and depth of this relationship. I'm not talking of love in imagination, or love of people. I'm talking of love in action . . . It is an attraction of polarities: one polarity seeks to merge with another to create a neutral state of mind.

–Yogi Bhajan

2 Then place one hand over the other at your heart center. Close your eyes, and meditate on your heart. Go deep within to the center of your being. Continue for 1½ minutes. When the time is up, inhale deeply and exhale deeply 3 times, then relax the posture, and thank your partner.

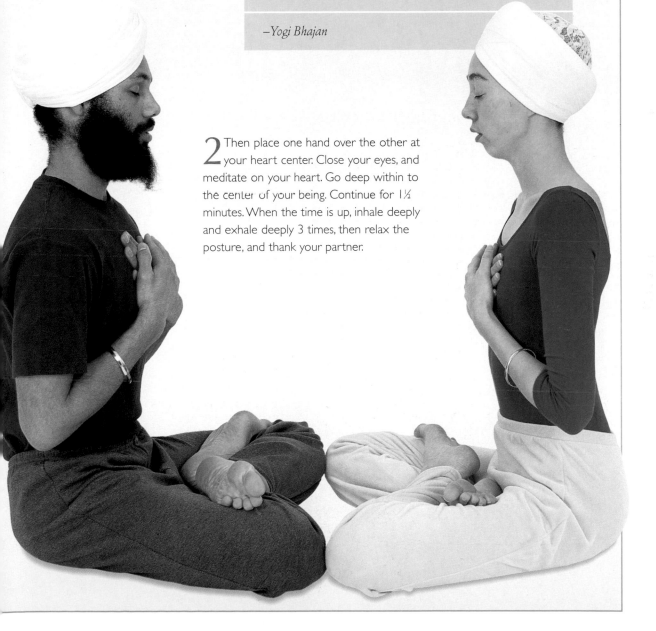

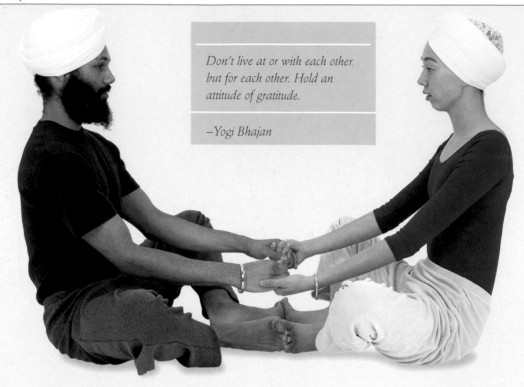

*Don't live at or with each other,
but for each other. Hold an
attitude of gratitude.*

—Yogi Bhajan

COUPLES KUNDALINI LOTUS

1 Sit across from each other, fairly close. Take the hands of your partner. With the legs outside of the arms, bend the knees and place the bottoms of your feet and your partner's feet together. Lean back slightly, straightening the arms. Slowly stretch the legs up straight to a 60° angle from the floor. Look into each other's eyes, projecting love and happiness. See yourself in the other person. Lift your partner's energy with your love, and realize that you two are one.

BACK ROLLS

Sit back to back with your partner. The lower spines are almost touching. The arms are relaxed at the sides. One partner bows forward as the other relaxes back onto the bowed back. Then smoothly reverse the roll. Exhale as you bend forward, and inhale as you bend backward. Keep the concentration on the breath and the third-eye point. Continue for 3 minutes. The vertebrae of your two backs should interlock like gears engaging.

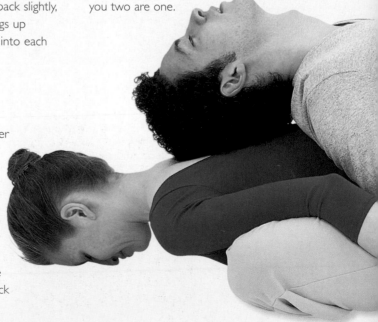

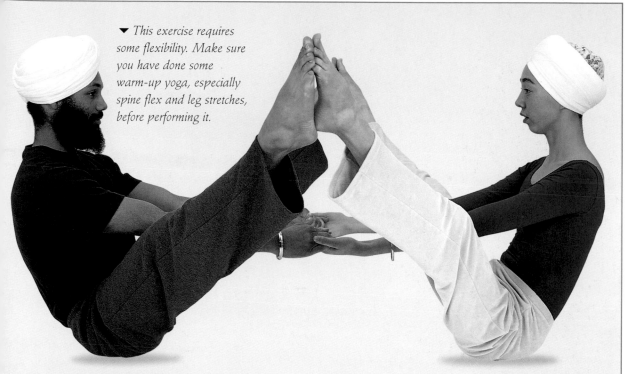

▼ *This exercise requires some flexibility. Make sure you have done some warm-up yoga, especially spine flex and leg stretches, before performing it.*

2 Continue for 3 minutes with either Breath of Fire or long deep breathing. (Decide before you start which type of breathing you will do. Both partners should do the same.) Inhale, exhale, and relax down.

Couples Kundalini Lotus helps to channel sexual energy and maintain potency. It brings both depth and lightness to your relationship.

▼ *This exercise relaxes the back and opens up the lower spine (while bowing) and upper spine (while bending back).*

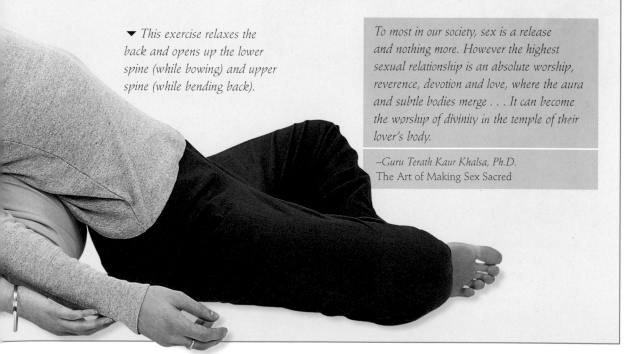

To most in our society, sex is a release and nothing more. However the highest sexual relationship is an absolute worship, reverence, devotion and love, where the aura and subtle bodies merge . . . It can become the worship of divinity in the temple of their lover's body.

–*Guru Terath Kaur Khalsa, Ph.D.*
The Art of Making Sex Sacred

MEDITATION TO RELEASE SUBCONSCIOUS FEAR

This is the *sa ta na ma* meditation for couples. Sit with a straight spine, back-to-back with your partner so that the lower spines are supporting each other. The middle spines should be slightly apart, and the upper spines may be touching. Sit on a firm pillow to adjust the difference in height if there is a great size disparity between you. Begin the *sa ta na ma* meditation on page 160. Continue for 2 to 5 minutes for each section. Coordinate yourselves so you are one voice.

This meditation has all the great benefits of individually practicing it, as well as the unified commitment of the couple to clearing the subconscious mind of fears, anger, insecurities, and other blocks to a happy, healthy relationship.

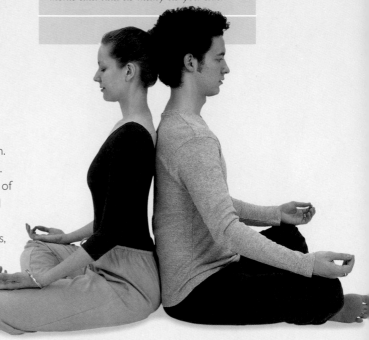

Don't count the deficiencies and demerits of your partner of life. Remember the merits and add as many as you can.

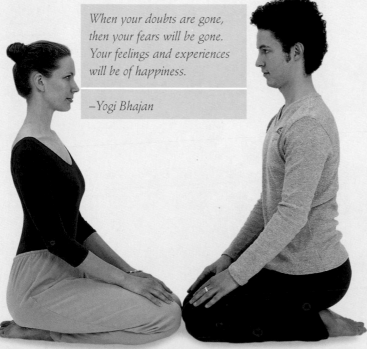

When your doubts are gone, then your fears will be gone. Your feelings and experiences will be of happiness.

—Yogi Bhajan

FOR RADIANT LOVE AND HEALTH

On the held inhalation and exhalation remember to suspend the breath in o out of the body with no pressure to the throat, chest, or face. Feel that you are circulating the prana, the vital energy, throughout your body and mind.

1 **Rock Pose** Sit, facing your partner, on the heels in Rock Pose with a straight spine. The hands are on the thighs, palms down. Look into each other's eyes without blinking. Radiate love and see yourself in your partner's eyes. Continue for 1 minute.

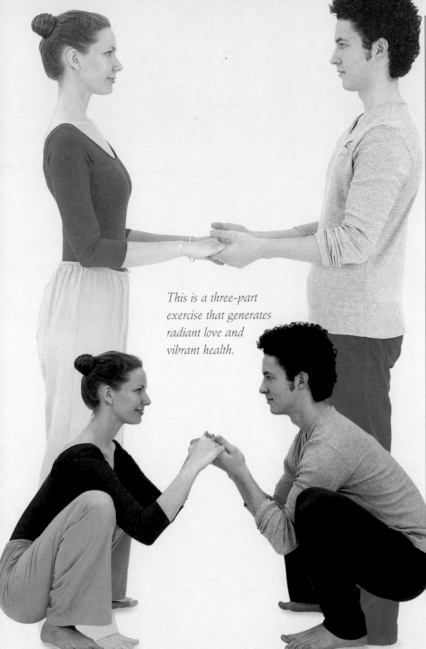

This is a three-part exercise that generates radiant love and vibrant health.

White Tantric Yoga

Tantra literally means "length and breadth." When cloth is woven there is a length (warp) and breadth (woof); that place where the opposites meet and merge is Tantra. The couple's yoga kriyas presented in the previous pages are similar to the meditative exercises practiced in White Tantric Yoga. As part of Kundalini Yoga, White Tantric Yoga is offered as a clarifying process for the male and female natures, enabling men and women to understand, appreciate, and discover bliss in their relationship to each other.

White Tantric Yoga courses are offered several times a year by 3HO. During the courses, partners sit opposite each other in a group meditation, and the subconscious fears and self-imposed limitations of the individual, the couple, and the entire group is filtered through Yogi Bhajan, who is the only living master of White Tantric Yoga. It has been said that Kundalini Yoga cleanses the unconscious mind, and White Tantric Yoga runs a river of love through it (see "Resources" section for information on White Tantric Yoga courses).

2 Crow Squats Stand up and face your partner. Place your feet shoulder-width apart and take hands with your partner. Begin crow squats in the following manner: Inhale standing up and hold the breath in for 5 to 10 seconds. Exhale and squat together, bringing the buttocks close to the ground. Keep the feel flat on the ground, if possible. Hold the exhalation out for 5 to 10 seconds while in squatting position. Then inhale, stand up, and repeat the sequence. Go up and down together, continuing to look into each other's eyes with radiant love. Continue for a total of 5 held inhalations and exhalations.

3 Rock Pose Lastly, face your partner sitting in Rock Pose on the heels again. Inhale and hold the breath in, then exhale and hold the breath out. Repeat 5 times. Then relax.

FAMILY YOGA

Perceiving children as big souls in little bodies, wise parents will dedicate themselves to helping their children connect with their innate wisdom and innocence. Yoga and meditation for the whole family are some of the best spiritual tools toward that end. Establishing family yoga and meditation time can start and end a day with peace and clarity. In the morning, yoga sets the "wavelength" for the day. In the evening, yoga wraps up a day with peaceful harmony. Taking a break in the middle of the day can also be the perfect time for settling into some yoga with your children.

Children can be great participants in yoga at any age, from babies on up to adolescence. One of the most essential requirements of children's yoga is that it has to be fun. Combine your own creativity with the resources provided at the end of the book. (See the "Resources" section for information on children's yoga books.)

GUIDELINES FOR CHILDREN'S YOGA

These are general guidelines. Be flexible when applying them to the temperament and abilities of individual children. Start with the shortest times given for beginners.

Please note that while the energy stimulated in Breath of Fire and the body locks is perfect for the adult body system, children should not practice these until they are in their teens.

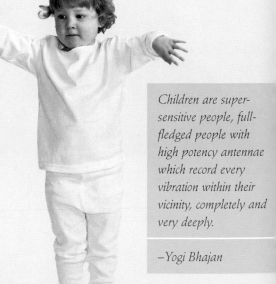

Children are super-sensitive people, full-fledged people with high potency antennae which record every vibration within their vicinity, completely and very deeply.

—Yogi Bhajan

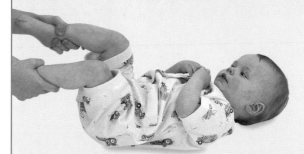

Babies and Crawlers Gently "bicycle" legs and cross arms closed, open, up, and down. Bundle the child in a light blanket and gently roll back to front, front to back. Chant and sing mantras and affirmations and smile with them.

Walkers and Toddlers Practice imaginative exercises like imitating animals (cobra, bear walk) and objects (washing machine). Do partner yoga to keep child involved. Perform each exercise for 15 to 30 seconds. Chant and sing for 1 minute of meditation.

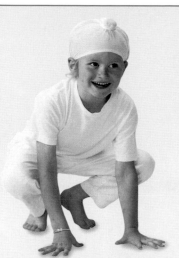

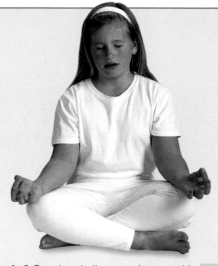

◀ Give the child yogic information to inspire. Meditate for 5 to ll minutes

Ages 3–5 years Practice imaginative exercises like imitating animals (Frog Hops, Seal Pose) and objects (Wheel Pose). Perform each exercise for 30 seconds to 1 minute. Children at this age can meditate silently or sing for 1 to 3 minutes.

Ages 6–8 Practice similar exercises as with preschoolers, but make them more challenging and less reliant on imagination. Give the child yogic information, to inspire. Perform each exercise for 1 minute. Meditate for 3 to 5 minutes.

Yoga for children is a mindful, active "play" that helps to:

• Increase self-awareness and self-confidence
• Strengthen bodies and physical coordination
• Promote focused mind and self-discipline
• Encourage awareness of the spirit
• Balance the brain and connect to the neutral mind

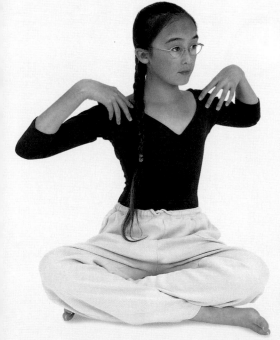

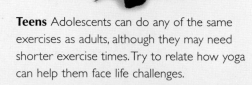

Ages 9–12 Children at this age can perform many of the same exercises as adults, but for shorter times (1 to 2 minutes). They may want to challenge themselves by timing their held poses. Give the child yogic information, to inspire. Meditate for 5 to ll minutes.

Teens Adolescents can do any of the same exercises as adults, although they may need shorter exercise times. Try to relate how yoga can help them face life challenges.

CHAPTER 9

HEALING
FOODS

Before there were pills, surgery, and medicine, there were healing foods. In ancient times, before the development of modern science, people in their simple wisdom looked to the food they ate as the source of their continued good health and as a cure for ailments. Food was their medicine. They learned the principles of healthful eating, and discovered the hidden properties of common foods and herbs, which could cleanse their bodies internally, correct imbalances that brought disease, and even heal damaged tissue.

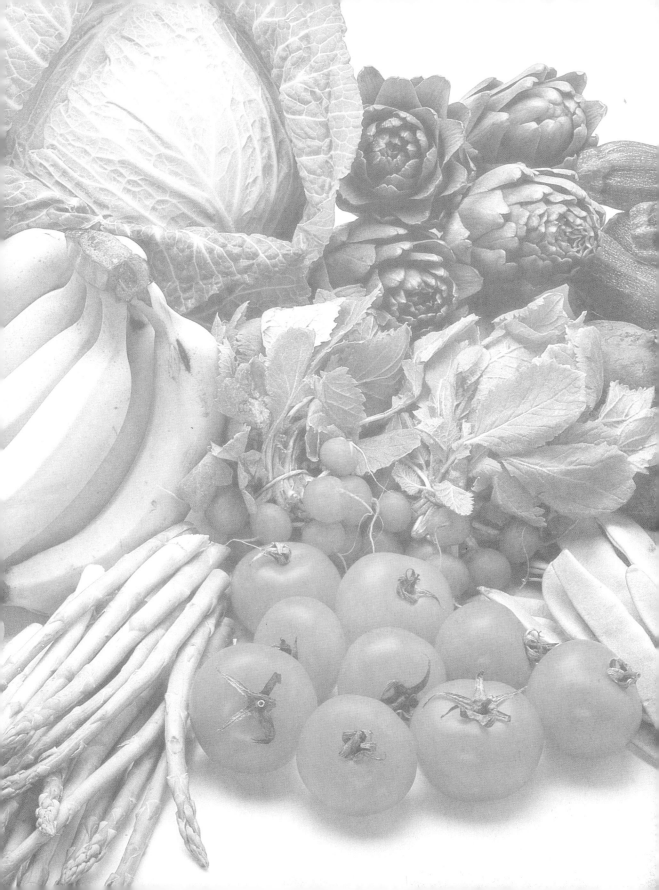

HEALING FOODS

Using food as medicine takes self-discipline, patience, and a commitment to preventative health care. It is one important way that we can reclaim responsibility for our own health and well-being. Along with balanced physical exercise such as the practice of yoga, and a positive attitude – which can be achieved through meditation – the food we eat is one of the three great pillars of total health.

Modern scientific research has confirmed that you can enhance the health of all the body's systems, and, in some cases, prevent problems from arising, through good nutrition. Additionally, as your practice of Kundalini Yoga deepens, you will naturally want your diet to reflect and enhance your clarity of consciousness.

The basics of a healthy diet include the following:

WATER

Water is the medium by which nutrients are transported to cells and wastes are removed. It is necessary for proper digestion, and helps to bring the emotions and nervous system into balance. Consuming six to eight glasses of water a day is recommended.

UNPROCESSED, WHOLE FOODS

Cold-pressed oils, natural sweeteners – such as maple syrup or honey – and whole grains are examples of foods that provide the nutrients that our bodies need. Always know what you are eating by reading the ingredient labels on packages, then judge if it will help or hinder the health of your body and mind.

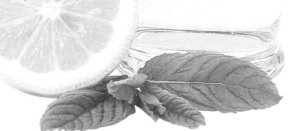

FRUITS, VEGETABLES, LEGUMES, AND GRAINS

Foods in their natural (preferably organic) state provide the vitamins, minerals, and protein that the body and mind need. The vegetarian diet supplies essential energy while maintaining a purity of body and mind. As a practitioner of Kundalini Yoga and someone concerned with the general well-being of your body, it is best to eliminate meat and eggs from the diet altogether, and to limit the intake of dairy products to organic yogurt and milk, or substitute soy or rice products for dairy. Not only will you feel physically and mentally fit, but you will also be practicing *ahimsa*, the sanskrit word for non-violence, toward animals, and in a larger sense, toward the entire planetary environment

On the subtle level, the yogic science teaches that food is nourishing in proportion to the amount of prana, life energy, that it embodies. Fresh, whole foods, prepared with mindful awareness, contain the maximum amount of prana. In India, the master cook is really a holistic healer, feeding not only the body but also the mind and spirit. While the ingredients in these dishes are believed to have curative properties in and of themselves, equally important is the love and positivity with which they are prepared and served. Singing, chanting, and consciously relaxing during the preparation and serving of a meal infuses the food with vitality and peace-giving properties. Taking a few moments to meditate and give thanks for the meal, then eating in appreciation, slowly savoring each bite, produces maximum spiritual, mental, and physical nourishment.

Most of the foods included here are based on the yogic system of cooking for health. The traditional yogic diet is purely lacto-vegetarian (fruits, vegetables, grains and milk products). It is naturally low in fats, cholesterol, and uric acid. The following foods and recipes have been time-tested for hundreds, even thousands, of years.

"Simple vegetarian food is referred to in Indian scriptures as sattvic bhoj. Sattvas means pure essence. Bhoj means food. A person who eats sattvic food is likely to be more calm, mentally agile, and clear thinking than one who eats heavier foods. The hot spices used in Indian cooking are said to have a rajasic quality. This means that they stimulate sexual energy, which is also the drive to create and achieve. Rajasic foods, taken in moderate amounts, are considered to be useful for people who work, or who practice Kundalini Yoga or martial arts. Tamasic foods, such as animal products and alcoholic beverages, are said to dull the mind and lead to sloth and regressive behavior."

–Bibiji Inderjit Kaur
A Taste of India: Delicious Vegetarian Recipes for Body, Mind, and Spirit

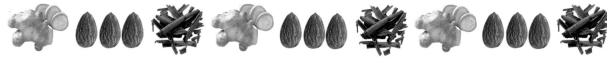

HEALING DRINKS

According to the yogic science of nutrition, it is best to drink at least an hour before or after eating, but not during a meal. This allows the digestive enzymes in the stomach to process the food without being diluted by liquids.

In all recipes, soy, rice or almond products may be used in place of dairy.

GOLDEN MILK

Turmeric, a root that is ground into a bright yellow powder, is one of the main ingredients in curry powder. Current research indicates that turmeric may be of value in preventing diabetes and cancer. Turmeric is best known as a lubricant for the joints. It is also excellent for the skin and for the mucous membranes, especially the female reproductive organs. It should always be cooked for at least 5 minutes in water or oil before using. Batches of the cooked solution can be stored in the refrigerator for up to a month, and taken out for use in recipes such as Golden Milk.

This very tasty drink is wonderful for the spine, lubricates the joints, and helps to break up calcium deposits.

¼-⅓ teaspoon turmeric
⅓ cup water
8 ounces milk, dairy or non-dairy
1 tablespoon raw almond oil
honey to taste

Boil turmeric in water for about 8 minutes. If too much water boils away, add a little more. Add milk and almond oil. When mixture boils, remove from heat and add honey. Makes 1-1½ cups of Golden Milk.

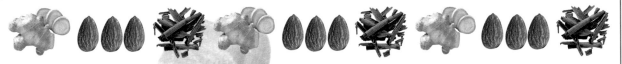

YOGI TEA

Health-promoting, delicious, soothing, and a great coffee substitute, the benefits of Yogi Tea would fill pages. In the science of yogic foods, the spices used in this tea are said to have the following properties:

Black pepper – a blood purifier
Cardamom pods – a digestive aid
Cloves – beneficial to the nervous system
Cinnamon – strengthens the bones
Ginger root – healing for colds and flu, and increases energy

The milk in this tea helps in the easy assimilation of the spices. A pinch of black tea acts as an alloy for all the ingredients, creating just the right chemical balance. Diluted with water or extra milk, it helps greatly with teething discomfort in young children. Yogi Tea can be made from scratch or it can be purchased as a mix. (See "Resources") It will store in the refrigerator for up to a week with milk and longer for the clear tea.

To 2 quarts of water, add the following:
15 whole cloves
20 green cardamom pods (crushed slightly)
15 black peppercorns
5 2-inch sticks of cinnamon, or equivalent in shorter lengths
8 slices ginger root
Boil gently, covered, for 30 to 40 minutes (adding water as it evaporates), then add:
½ teaspoon black tea
3-4 cups of milk (according to preference)

Bring to a boil. Turn off and add honey to taste. Strain and serve. Makes 2-3 quarts.

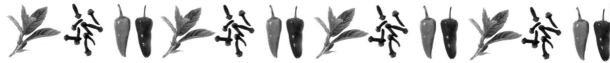

WEIGHT-LOSS TEA

This tea has been used to dissolve fatty tissue. Drink 2 to 3 glasses per day for this purpose. Weight-loss tea also improves the beauty and youthfulness of the skin, cleanses the mucous membrane of the colon, and is an excellent source of Vitamin C.

Black salt and tamarind can be found in Asian stores. Black salt, a superb, health-giving food, has been used as a cancer preventative. It has a strong taste, and even stronger smell, so use just a pinch. Tamarind is a sweet-sour tropical fruit, and is sold as a paste with or without the seeds.

¼-⅓ fresh or dried mint leaves
2 cups cumin seeds
1 tablespoon fresh or frozen tamarind
¼ teaspoon black salt
4 lemons, quartered
½ tablespoon black pepper
3 quarts of water

Combine all the ingredients in a pot and bring to a boil. Lower the heat and cook covered at a low boil for several hours. This is necessary to draw the extract from the cumin seeds. Replace water if it begins to evaporate. Strain and serve hot or cold. The ingredients can be reused to make more tea, just add fresh lemons. Tea can be stored for up to a week in the refrigerator. Makes 2½-3 quarts.

JALAPEÑO MILK

At the first sign of a cold or flu, Jalapeño Milk is the remedy to head off sickness. Be careful–it is hot! Start with the minimum quantity of jalapeños. It is helpful to keep frozen jalapeños in a plastic bag in the freezer. When frozen, they are easier to chop, their odor is less harsh, and the juice does not get on the fingers.

In blender, combine:
2-5 fresh or frozen jalapeño chiles
8 ounces milk

A tip for drinking Jalapeño Milk: It is not as hot when sipped through a straw.

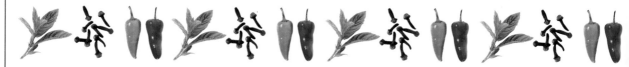

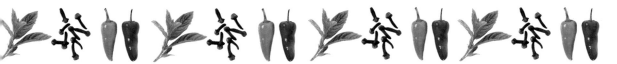

MANGO LASSI

A lassi (lussee) is a yogurt-based drink, wonderful for breakfast or a snack. Mangos have been used as a remedy for liver disorders, menstrual problems, and general digestive problems. In combination with fresh–preferably homemade–yogurt, which contains beneficial bacteria, a mango lassi isa tonic for the entire digestive tract. Please note that mangos are acidic, and need to be balanced by combining wih diary products.

2 cups plain yogurt
2 medium, very ripe mangos, peeled and sliced
2-3 tablespoons maple syrup or honey
6 ice cubes, or ⅔ cup water
⅛ teaspoon rose water (optional, available at Asian stores,
adds a fragrant Indian touch)

Blend until smooth and creamy. Makes approximately 4 cups.

SESAME-GINGER MILK

This creamy drink is nourishing to the nervous system, and is especially healthful for the male sexual organs, stimulating the production of healthy sexual fluids.

¼ cup of sesame seeds
2 tablespoons coarsely chopped fresh ginger root
12 ounces milk
2 teaspoons honey or maple syrup

Blend at high speed until smooth and frothy. Makes about 2 cups.

GINGER TEA

At once calming to the nerves and energizing to the body and mind, ginger tea is good for everyone, and especially helpful for women during their monthly menses.

4 to 6 1/8-inch-thick slices of fresh ginger root (unpeeled is fine)
2 cups water
lemon juice and honey

Bring water to a boil and add ginger root slices. Boil until the water is light brown in color, about 15 minutes. Add fresh lemon juice and honey to taste. Milk may be substituted for lemon juice

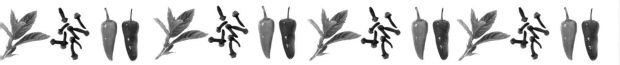

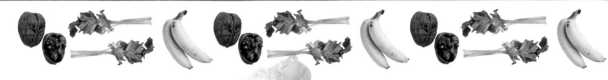

CARDAMOM-FENNEL TEA

Both cardamom and fennel are digestive aids, so the combination of the two makes for a powerful digestive helper.

4 cups of water
5 black cardamom pods (can be found at Asian
stores – if substituting green cardamom pods, use 10)
1 tablespoon fennel seeds

Boil all ingredients together, covered, for 20 minutes to ½ hour, until the water turns brown. Add more water if needed. Add a small amount of milk and honey at the end. Makes 2½-3 cups.

BANANA ICE CREAM OR MILK SHAKE

Bananas are one of nature's perfect foods. This recipe uses frozen bananas, which is a wonderful way to keep bananas that are getting over-ripe. Just freeze them with or without peels. If with peels, run hot water over the bananas when you want to use them, and the skins will peel off easily. Do not remove the stringy part underneath the peel. It will blend right in, and is a mineral-rich part of the banana.

In a blender, combine:
2 frozen bananas, broken into pieces
½-⅔ cup dairy or non-dairy milk
(use twice as much liquid if making a shake)

Blend together until creamy. For ice cream, add chopped walnuts, pecans, or carob chips, if desired.

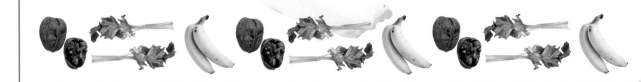

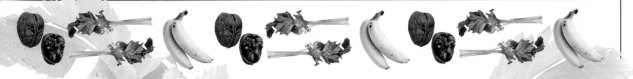

HEALTHY DRINKS FOR CHILDREN

Children have different dietary needs than adults, and what might be good for an adult may not always be suitable for a child. Following are recipes well suited to their developing digestive systems.

CELERY RAISIN DRINK

This drink helps to calm and relax children.

2 stalks of celery
1 handful of raisins

Place the raisins in a pan and cover with 1 or 2 inches of purified water. Bring to a boil, and cook for a few minutes until the water is colored by the raisins. Remove from heat and strain the raisin water into a cup. While the raisins are boiling, put the celery through a juicer. Mix the two together, cool, and serve. For very young children, dilute by half with water.

DATE MILK

The soothing, delicious taste of date milk helps wean babies from breastfeeding while providing nourishment to replace the mother's milk. Date milk is a very nutritious, youth-maintaining beverage for people of all ages. It gives energy to the body, and helps to ward off colds. Great when recovering from fevers or flu.

4 ounces water
8 ounces milk
6 dates, sliced in half

Simmer ingredients together on low heat for 20 minutes, or until the milk is a pinkish color and the dates are disintegrating. Stir occasionally. Strain before serving. Makes 1 cup.

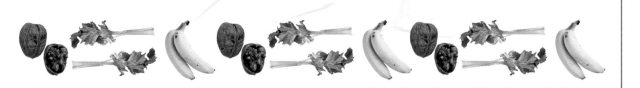

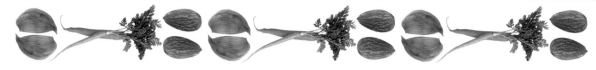

ANCIENT YOGIC RECIPES

GHEE

In the medical writings of ancient India, ghee is highly regarded as both a nutrient and a preservative for food and medicine. It is also known as clarified butter, because the impurities have been removed through the heating process. Anything cooked in ghee will retain its freshness and nutritional value much longer. Stored in a sealed container, ghee will keep 3-4 months without refrigeration in mild temperatures. It is low in cholesterol and contains no salt.

Simmer unsalted butter for 10 to 20 minutes in a heavy-bottomed pot or crock-pot over a medium-low heat until a crust forms on top. Skim off the crust and strain the golden liquid that remains into a container; do not allow the sediment in the bottom to pour in.

ALMONDS

The almond is a wonderful nut. Its oil is beneficial both internally and externally for the skin. Almonds are an excellent source of protein. They are a good source of manganese, phosphorus, and potassium. It is often best to remove the astringent outside skin before eating.

To blanch almonds, soak in pure water overnight. Strain and pour warm (not boiling) water over them, as you slip the skins off. Store unused almonds covered in water in the refrigerator.

For Women

 During the first few mornings of a woman's menstrual cycle and during the first 40 days after giving birth, she can gain energy and avoid cramping by sautéeing a handful of unpeeled almonds then, adding a little honey at the end. This combination of foods rejuvenates the female reproductive organs, and is one of the few times almonds should be eaten with the skins on.

ALMOND OIL

Two tablespoons of raw almond oil taken in food or drink each day will help lower cholesterol, reduce body fat and hunger, cleanse the body of toxins, and keep the skin healthy and lustrous. Good on vegetables or grains.

TRINITY ROOTS

Onions, garlic, and ginger are considered by yogis to be the "Trinity Roots." While each of these roots is beneficial when taken alone, cooking them together causes them to interact, amplifying their effect on the body. Onions purify the blood, garlic boosts the immune system, and ginger aids the nervous and reproductive systems.

MASALA

The word masala means blend, and this masala is a yogic blend of spices and the Trinity Roots.

Basic masala: Sauté one onion in canola oil. After 1 minute, add 1 tablespoon of turmeric. After 5 minutes, add 2 tablespoons of grated (peel before grating) ginger. After 5 more minutes, add 3 cloves of minced garlic. Cook until all is soft and blended. Add vegetables or beans and salt, soy sauce, or Bragg's Liquid Aminos. Note: Bragg's Liquid Aminos is a soy sauce substitute that has no added salt. It can be found in natural food stores.

WHEATBERRIES

The whole wheat "berry," from which wheat flour is milled, is an excellent food when boiled until tender. It cleans the intestinal tract, gives strong teeth and gums, beautifies the skin, and can help to prevent stomach disorders, including cancer.

Basic Cooked Wheatberries: Soak ½ cup wheatberries overnight in 2 cups purified water. Drain, and cook on medium-high heat in 2½ to 3 cups of water. Cook until the wheat is puffed up and tender, about 1 hour. Wheatberries can be cooked overnight in a crock-pot. Use as a breakfast cereal blended with milk and honey, or as a main dish made with masala.

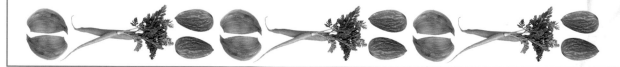

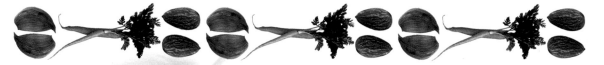

BASMATI RICE

This naturally white rice is revered throughout Asia as a sacred food. It is also grown in Mexico. Basmati is a fragrant, high-quality white rice that is not milled or polished, which can strip away most of the vitamin and mineral content of rice. Basmati rice is abundant in B vitamins, iodine, and high-quality protein, and is easily assimilated. Brown rice, although rich in vitamins, can be hard to digest unless cooked for a very long time. Basmati rice cooks in a 2 to 1 ratio with water in about 20 minutes.

KICHEREE

Kicheree is a very digestible, balanced protein, ideal for rebuilding strength during and after illness. It is a soothing, healthful addition to a basic vegetarian diet. For quick heat-up cook a larger batch and store in the refrigerator for up to a week. Add more water for a soupier consistency, less for a stew-like consistency.

½ cup mung beans (washed and
picked through for small stones)
1 cup basmati rice
2½ quarts water (more or less
according to your taste)
5 cloves garlic, finely minced
¼ cup ginger, finely minced
1 large onion, finely chopped
3 cups vegetables, finely chopped: carrots,
potatoes, zucchini, green beans
¼-½ teaspoon each cumin seeds,
cracked red chili, and black pepper
Bragg's Liquid Amino Acids or soy sauce to taste
½ cup ghee

Cook mung beans on medium high until beans begin to break open. Meanwhile, in another pot, add chopped onions, garlic, and ginger to the water. Let the water boil. Add chopped vegetables. Add Bragg's or soy sauce and spices. After mung beans are ready, strain them if there is an excess of liquid (otherwise add the liquid to the rice as well), and add them into the pot along with the rice. Cook until all ingredients are blended, stirring often. As the last step before serving, stir in the ghee. Serves 4 to 6.

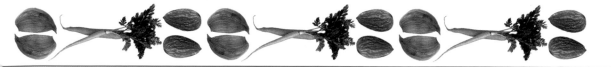

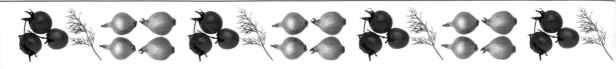

YOGURT CURRY

To soothe and strengthen the nervous system, and to please the palate.

1 cup basmati rice
3 cups chopped mixed vegetables
¼ cup minced ginger
2 cloves garlic, minced
2 small onions, finely chopped
½ cup ghee
1½ teaspoon crushed Yogi Tea spices (see "Resources" for Yogi Tea products)
1 tablespoon turmeric
¼ teaspoon oregano seeds
½ teaspoon cumin seeds
¼ teaspoon ground black pepper
1 teaspoon garam masala
1 cup yogurt (homemade preferred, or organic)
¼ cup besan (chickpea flour from Asian store)

Steam chopped mixed vegetables until firm but tender. Make basmati rice according to recipe above. Blend yogurt and besan flour with 1 cup of water until smooth. Sauté spices in ghee until golden brown. Add chopped onion, garlic, and ginger. Cook slowly until mixture is blended. Stir in yogurt-flour mixture. Simmer until sauce thickens. Serve over rice and steamed vegetables. Serves 4.

POTENT POTATOES

4 Russet baking potatoes
½ cup canola oil
3 medium onions, chopped
3 tablespoons ginger, minced
2 teaspoons garlic, minced
1 teaspoon crushed red chilies or cayenne pepper (more or less to taste)
½ teaspoon ground cloves
1 teaspoon cardamom powder or seeds, or 3 cardamom pods
½ teaspoon ground cinnamon
⅓ cup tamari (soy) sauce
½ pint cottage cheese
4 slices mild cheese, cut in half

Bake potatoes at 400°F until soft on the inside and crispy on the outside, approximately 45 minutes. Meanwhile, heat the oil in a skillet and add onions. Sauté for approximately 10 minutes, then add ginger. Cook until well-done, then add garlic and spices. Add more oil or water if the mixture sticks. Cook until all the spices and root vegetables melt together. Add tamari. Turn off heat.
Cut potatoes in half lengthwise when cool enough to handle. Scoop out insides, leaving enough potato in the shell so that it does not tear. Combine potato insides with onion mixture and add cottage cheese. Refill shells, forming mounds on top. Cover each shell with a slice of cheese and broil or bake until melted and golden brown. Makes 8 halves.

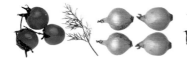
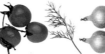

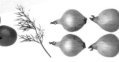

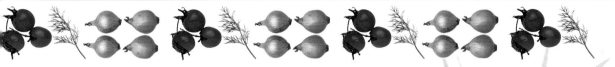

SOUP OF LIFE

Onions, garlic, and ginger are the three roots of life. Basil, dill, and oregano are the three herbs of life. Pepper is for the blood, ajawan (oregano seed) is known for its healing properties and as a disease preventative. Turmeric is for the spine and joints. The broth of this soup is very invigorating, and keeps well, getting tastier in the next few days after it is made.

¾ cup sesame or canola oil

2-3 onions sliced thin

¼ cup minced ginger root

2 teaspoons turmeric

1 teaspoon black pepper

1 tablespoon caraway seeds

½ teaspoon ajawan (oregano seeds)

Can be found in Asian stores

1 tablespoon poppy seeds

1 tablespoon celery seeds

1 tablesoon garam masala (an Asian ground spice combination)

2 to 3 ripe tomatoes, steamed, peeled and chopped

3 tablespoons basil

1 tablespoon dill weed

1 tablespoon oregano

1 tablespoon tarragon

1-2 diced potatoes (unpeeled to maintain the acid/alkaline balance of the potato)

2 to 3 carrots, diced

4 cups chopped assorted vegetables

soy sauce, Bragg's Liquid Amino Acids, or sea salt

10 cloves garlic, minced

In the bottom of a soup pot, heat the sesame or canola oil on medium-high heat. Add onions and ginger. There should be enough oil so that they do not scorch or stick. Make a "pool" in the center of the onion-ginger mixture, and add turmeric, pepper, caraway, ajawan, poppy seeds, celery seeds, and garam masala. Sauté for 2 minutes, then mix well with onions. Add tomatoes and herbs. Add 3 quarts water and the vegetables. Bring to a boil, then simmer over medium heat for about 1 hour. Add salt or soy sauce and garlic, and simmer 5 minutes longer. Serves 10.

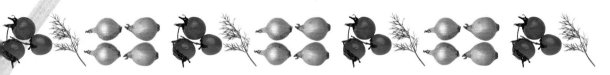

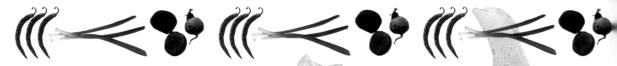

BEETS

Beets cleanse the liver and digestive tract. To help your body do its own inner cleaning, eat only beets for 1 week in the spring or fall. Beet juice is best taken in small quantities and in combination with other juices. Beets aid in the treatment of hemorrhoids, eliminating toxins from the body, and regulating the blood sugar. Cut the greens from the beets and steam or sautée with onions. Steam the beets until soft. Once the beets are soft, run cold water over them as you rub them in your hands. The peels will slide off. Cooked beets can be stored for at least 1 week in the refrigerator.

BEETS AND CARROTS

5 medium beets, cooked, peeled, and grated
6 organic carrots, peeled and grated
3 spring onions, finely chopped
canola oil for sautéing
½ teaspoon rosemary
1 teaspoon chopped garlic
dash of pepper and salt
1 cup grated mild cheese (dairy or non-dairy)

Sauté onions and grated carrots in canola oil on medium heat for 5 minutes. Add garlic and spices and sauté for 5 minutes more. Add grated beets and toss lightly. Cover with cheese and turn heat to low, cooking until cheese is melted. Serves 4 to 6.

JALAPEÑO PANCAKES

In India, these are known for their healing properties for colds and the flu. They give you energy, too! This recipe has been adapted to Western tastes by substituting ⅓ pancake mix for the besan flour. The amount of spices can be cut by ¼ for those who like less-spicy food.

olive oil (or canola oil) for frying
⅔ cup besan (chickpea flour from Asian store)
⅓ cup multi-grain pancake mix
8-10 almonds, soaked in water overnight, peeled and halved
¼ cup finely minced or grated ginger
4 cloves of garlic, finely minced
1-2 large jalapeño peppers, finely minced
2 teaspoons coriander seed
½-1 teaspoon salt
½-1 teaspoon cracked red chilies
1 teaspoon ajawan (oregano) seed
½ teaspoon black pepper
1 teaspoon cumin seeds

Add water to besan and pancake batter to make a good pancake consistency. Add remaining ingredients, except oil. In skillet, heat small amount of oil. Add large spoonfuls of batter and spread evenly in a circle. Fry like pancakes, browning on both sides. Serve with yogurt. Serves 4 to 6.

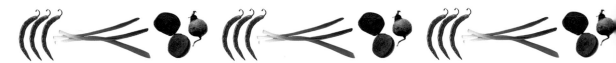

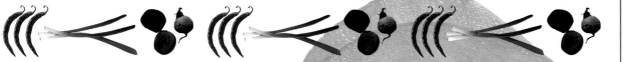

NATURAL SALAD

This is an unusual salad, containing no lettuce but lots of pleasing taste. The use of fresh parsley adds rich minerals, helps in cleansing the kidneys and regulating the calcium balance in the body, and has been shown to be helpful in treating diabetes. Kelp, a dried seaweed, is high in minerals and iodine, which is beneficial to the health of the thyroid gland. Celery aids the nerves, and sunflower seeds add high-quality protein. The finer the ingredients are diced and grated, the better.

1 cup grated carrots
1 cup grated mild cheese (or soy cheese)
2 cups bread crumbs (or small bread cubes)
½ cup raw sunflower seeds
1 cup diced celery
1 cup finely chopped parsley
¼-½ cup finely diced onion

Toss the above ingredients together in a bowl. Combine the following ingredients in a blender to make the dressing:

½ cup sesame or almond oil
1-2 tablespoons of Braggs Liquid Amino Acids, or soy sauce
1 tablespoon honey
3 tablespoons lemon juice
2 teaspoon basil
1 teaspoon sage
1 teaspoon kelp
½ cup water

Toss the salad with the dressing. Serves 6.

RATATOUILLE

Each of the vegetables in this dish have specific healing properties: zucchini is for good elimination and healthy skin; red peppers contain copious amounts of vitamin C, the anti-stress vitamin; and eggplant is considered to be the most powerful food for a woman, energizing and soothing.

1 onion, chopped finely
1 medium eggplant, peeled, or 8 small Asian eggplants (unpeeled is okay)
3 medium zucchini
1 sweet red pepper
¼ cup olive oil
1 cup diced tomatoes (fresh or canned)
½ tablespoon each of garlic, basil, oregano, dill
½ teaspoon black pepper
salt to taste

If using regular-sized eggplant, cut into finger-sized sticks and steam for 5 to 8 minutes. Remove any large clusters of seeds after steaming. If using Asian eggplant, slice in thin rounds and do not steam. Quarter zucchini lengthwise and cut into 2-inch sticks. Sauté onion in olive oil for 10 minutes, then add spices and garlic and cook a few minutes more. Add tomatoes, eggplant, and zucchini. Cook until vegetable are soft but firm. Serve with couscous or basmati rice. Serves 4 to 6.

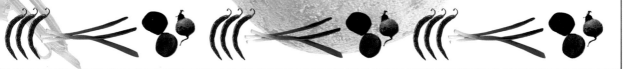

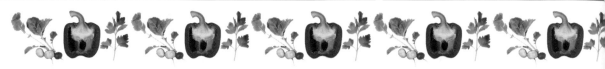

HEALTH-GIVING TOFU

Tofu, one of the most versatile protein foods, has been a staple in parts of Asia for over 2,000 years and is now well-known in the West. Also called bean curd, tofu is made by curdling the mild white "milk" of the soybean. It is high in protein, low in calories, fats, and carbohydrates, and contains no cholesterol. Recent medical news shows that soy protein can help prevent heart disease, breast cancer, and prostate cancer, ease menopause symptoms, and help in diabetes and digestive disorders. For those who are lactose intolerant, or want a substitute for meat or dairy, tofu is the logical and delicious choice. Always rinse tofu before using, and keep any remaining pieces covered in water in the refrigerator. To minimize the gas-producing quality of tofu, always cook tofu before eating, covering it in a bit of lemon juice. As a rule, use firm tofu for slicing and dicing and soft tofu for blending.

BAKED TOFU

Use I block (I pound) of firm or extra-firm tofu. Rinse and lightly squeeze out excess water. Slice ¼ to ½ inch thick. Thin slices will quickly bake into chewy, hard tofu, thicker slices will yield soft tofu, depending on how long it is baked. It is recommended to use a glass baking pan, but a baking sheet can also be used. Cover the bottom of the pan with canola oil; water can be used in place of oil. Sprinkle lemon juice over the tofu. After topping with Braggs Liquid or soy sauce (tamari), you may bake as is or add any combination of the following: herbs, garlic/onion powder or flakes, salt-free seasonings, nutritional yeast flakes, sugar-free barbecue sauce, Japanese condiments.
Bake for 20 to 40 minutes at 350°F to 375°F. The longer the cooking time, the crispier or chewier the texture will be.

MARINATED TOFU

Slice tofu as described above. Cover bottom of glass baking pan lightly with oil. Marinate for at least 2 hours in a mixture of ¼ cup soy sauce, ¼ cup water, and I tablespoon finely grated peeled ginger. Garlic may be finely minced and added to the marinade as well. Flip tofu once while marinating. Bake at 350°F for 30 minutes, adding water as necessary. Serve with stir-fried vegetables.

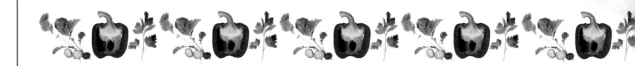

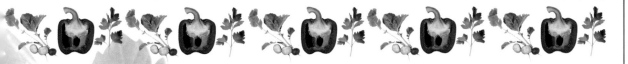

TOFU SALAD

The texture of the grated baked tofu in this dish is similar to chicken or tuna salad.

Slice 1½ pounds of firm tofu approximately ½-inch thick. Lightly sprinkle with lemon juice, and bake in a lightly oiled baking dish at 375°F until medium hard, about 20 to 25 minutes. Grate when cooled.

Meanwhile, mix in one bowl:

3 celery sticks, finely diced

⅔ cup grated radishes, carrots, and/or raw zucchini

½ sweet red pepper, finely chopped

⅔ dill pickles, finely chopped

Add the grated tofu to the ingredients of the first bowl, and mix well. Add the dressing, and serve with crackers or with lettuce on bread. Serves 4.

Mix the dressing separately:

¼-½ cup eggless, sugarless mayonnaise (can be found at natural food stores)

2-3 tablespoon prepared mustard

1 teaspoon lemon juice

½ teaspoon sea salt

½ teaspoon black pepper

TOFU SPREAD

Both tofu and sesame seeds are high in calcium and protein, and both are used in this dish. Tahini is sesame seed paste, and can be found at supermarkets, natural food, or middle-eastern stores. Nutritional yeast flakes have a cheesy taste, are high in B vitamins, and are found at natural food stores.

1 pound firm tofu, rinsed and squeezed of excess water

1–2 sticks celery, finely diced

1 scallion, finely chopped

⅛ cup fresh parsley

⅛ cup either diced sweet red pepper or finely grated carrots

Steam tofu for 5 to 10 minutes in a steamer to release gas-producing qualities. Squeeze any remaining water from the tofu once again. Crumble and mash tofu with the above ingredients.

In a separate bowl, mix:

1 tablespoon lemon juice

⅓–½ cup eggless, sugarless mayonnaise

1½ tablespoons nutritional yeast flakes

½–1 teaspoon salt

1 teaspoon vegetable seasoning such as Jensen's or Spike

2 tablespoons sesame tahini

Combine tofu mixture with mayonnaise mixture. Serve with crackers or vegetable sticks, or as a sandwich spread. Makes approximately 2½ cups.

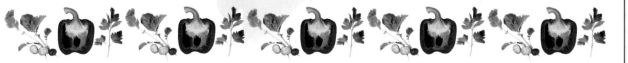

GLOSSARY

Adi Mantra (AA-dee MUN-traa) Literally, primal or original mantra. Refers to the mantra used to tune-in before doing Kundalini Yoga.

Affirmation Positive statement that, when spoken, retrains the mind.

Amrit Vela (AHM-rit VEH-la) Literally, the ambrosial time. Refers to the early hours of the morning before dawn.

Amritsar (AHM-rit-sahr) Literally, the tank of nectar. Refers to a place in Northern India where resides the Golden Temple and its healing waters.

Apana (ah-PAH-na) The outgoing, cleansing breath of life; the eliminative energy.

Arcline The part of the energy field which extends out from the hairline level, sometimes called a halo.

Aura The field of energy that surrounds and interpenetrates the entire body and is considered to be the 8th chakra.

Bandha (BUN-dhaa) Body lock formed by pulling internal muscles.

Bij (Beej) Literally, seed. Sat Nam is called the bij or seed mantra.

Brosa (BROH-sa) The element of trust.

Buddhi mudra (BUHD-hi MOO-dra) Hand position for communication.

Chakra (CHAHK-ra) Literally, circle. There are seven energy centers of consciousness associated with the seven nerve centers of the body.

Electromagnetic energy field The field of energy surrounding and moving through a living being.

Gian mudra (GHEE-ahn MOO-dra) Hand position for wisdom.

Hatha (HAAT-ha) Yogic path primarily utilizing postures, and emphasizing development of the human will.

Higher Triangle The second four chakras of the body, associated with the heart, throat, third-eye point, and crown center.

Hydrotherapy The yogic science of using cold water and massage to revitalize and heal the body.

Ida (EE-dah) Left nerve channel which relates to the left nostril and moon (negative pole) energy.

Jalandhara Bandha (JAA-lund-HAR-a BUN-dhaa) The neck lock.

Japa (JAA-pa) Literally, to resound the mantra. To repeat a sound vibration as meditation.

Khalsa (KHAAL-sah) Literally, "pure one." Refers to the pure spirit which is every human's birthright.

Kirtan (KEER-tan) Spiritual, or sacred music.

Kriya (KREE-ya) Literally, a completed action. A particular yogic posture or series of postures linked to mantra and breath to produce a particular effect.

Kundalini (Kuhn-da-LIN-ee) From the root word, kundal, meaning literally, "the lock of hair of the beloved." It refers to the coiled energy which is the creative potential of the individual.

Laya Yoga (LAY-ah) A form of meditation that uses rhythmic patterns of mantra and locks.

Lower Triangle The first three chakras of the body, associated with the rectum, sexual organs, and navel center.

Maha Bandha (Maa-haa BUN-dhaa) The great lock, formed by pulling all three body locks at once.

Mala (Maa-laa) A string of beads used as an aid in repeating a mantra.

Maya (MY-ya) The illusion of the reality of sensory experience of one's self and the world around us.

Mantra (MUN-tra) Literally, mind-guiding sound. Sound current that tunes and controls mental vibration.

Mudra (MOO-dra) Yogic hand position.

Mul Bandha (MOOL BUN-dhaa) The root lock. The most commonly used lock in Kundalini Yoga.

Nabhi (NAA-bhee) The navel center, seat of physical well-being.

Numerology Can be referred to as Akara or Tantric numerology, this is the yogic system for understanding how the ten bodies work in our individual lives.

Padmasana (Pud-MAA-suh-nah) Lotus sitting pose.

Pingala (Pin-GAHL-a) Right nerve channel which relates to the right nostril and sun (positive pole) energy.

Prana (PRAA-na) The subtle life force, carried to us by the air we breath.

Pranayam (PRAA-na-yum) Yogic system of breathing exercises.

Ram Das (Raam Daas) Literally, servant of God. Can refer to the fourth of the Sikh masters who was known for service and humility.

Sadhana (SAAD-na) Daily spiritual practice, especially in the early morning hours before dawn.

Samadhi (sah-MAAD-ee) The state of consciousness in which the mind is merged in the blissful absorption of the Infinite.

Sat Nam (Sut Naam) Literally, Truth-Name, or Truth Manifested.

Sanskrit (SAAN-skrit) The ancient and sacred language of India.

Shabd (SHAH-bid) Literally, the sacred word, and the sound current it generates.

Shuni mudra (SHOO-ni MOO-dra) Hand position for patience and self-discipline.

Shushmana (SHUSH-man-a) Central spinal channel.

Sitali breath (Si-TAAL-ee) Cooling breath that relaxes.

Sukasana (sukh-AAS-a-nah) Easy sitting pose.

Surya mudra (SOOR-ya MOO-dra) Literally "the sun," hand position for energy.

Tapa (TUP-ah) The inner psychic "heat" of the prana which comes from repeating a mantra (japa).

Tattvas (TAAT-vaas) The five elements of which everything is composed; fire, air, earth, ether, and water.

Tenth Gate Another name for the crown (7th) chakra. Also called the "Thousand Petaled Lotus."

Third-eye point A point of concentration midway between the brows that relates to the individual's center of intuition. Also called the brow point, and sixth chakra.

Uddiyana Bhanda (Oo-di-YAAN-ah BUN-dhaa) The diaphragm lock.

Vajrasana (Vaaj-RAAS-an-ah) Sitting on the heels in rock pose.

Venus Lock A hand position used frequently in Kundalini yoga exercises.

White Tantric Yoga The yogic science of applied consciousness in regard to the union of opposites.

Yoga Literally, union. Refers to the union of body, mind, and spirit.

RESOURCES

RECOMMENDED BOOKS

KUNDALINI YOGA AND YOGIC TEACHINGS

Kundalini Yoga: The Flow of Eternal Power by Shakti Parwha Kaur Khalsa, Perigree, 1998

The Mind: Its Projections and Multiple Facets by Yogi Bhajan, Ph.D with Gurucharan Singh Khalsa, Ph.D., KRI, 1998

The Master's Touch by Yogi Bhajan, Ph. D.,KRI, 1997

The Teachings of Yogi Bhajan, Arcline, 1977

How to Know God by Swami Prabhavananda & Christopher Isherwood, Vedanta Press, 1981

Breathwalk by Yogi Bhajan, Ph.D. and Gurucharan Singh Khalsa, Ph.D., Broadway Books, 2000

Meditation for Absolutely Everyone by Subagh Singh Khalsa, Chas. Tuttle Co., 1994

The Art of Making Sex Sacred by Guru Terath Kaur Khalsa, Ph.D., Yogi Ji Press, 1998

Your Life is in Your Chakras by Gururattan Kaur Khalsa, Ph.D, Yoga Technology Press, 1994

Mala Meditation by Guru Kirn Kaur Khalsa, Sacred Gems, 1994

Sacred Sexual Bliss by Sat-Kaur Khalsa, Ed. D., Yogi Ji Press, 2000

Kundalini Yoga for Body, Mind and Beyond, by Ravi Singh, White Lion Press, 1989

Heal Your Back Now! by Nirvair Singh Khalsa (book and video), NSK Brokers, 1998

Akara Numerology by Nam Hari K. Khalsa, NHK Productions, 1998

Numerology As Taught By Yogi Bhajan, by Guruchander Singh Khalsa, Radiant Light Press, 1993

YOGIC HEALING ARTS

The Anatomy of Healing by Subagh Singh Khalsa, Chas. Tuttle Co, 1999

The Miracle of Healing Hands by Waheguru Singh Khalsa, D.C., Rishi Knot Pub., 1997

Brain Longevity by Dharma Singh Khalsa, M.D., Warner Books, 1999

Meditation as Medicine by Dharma Singh Khalsa, M.D., Simon & Schuster

The Pain Cure by Dharma Singh Khalsa M.D., Warner Books, 2000

The Ancient Art of Self-Healing by Siri Amir Singh Khalsa, D.C., Silverstreak Press, 1982

A Call to Women: The Healthy Breast Program and Workbook by Sat Dharam Kaur, N.D., Quarry Press, 1999

FOOD AND COOKING

The Golden Temple Vegetarian Cookbook, Arcline Pub. 1978

From Vegetables with Love by Siri Ved Kaur Khalsa, Arcline Pub. 1989

A Taste of India by Bibiji Inderjit Kaur, Arcline Pub. 1985

Foods for Health and Healing, KRI, 1983

Diet For a New America by John Robbins, H. J. Kramer, 1987

CHILDREN

Fly Like A Butterfly: Yoga for Children by Shakta Kaur Khalsa, Sterling Pub., 1998

The Five Fingered Family by Shakta Kaur Khalsa, Brookfield Reader, 2000

72 Stories of God, Good, and Goods by Yogi Bhajan, Harimandir Pub., 1989

Child's Play by Wahe Guru Kaur Khalsa (audio tape/CD)

WEBSITES

3ho.home.pages.de

AlzheimersPrevention.org

Brain-Longevity.com

breathwalk.com

brookfieldreader.com

childrensyoga.com

darshanyogastudio.com

healthybreastprogram.on.ca

interarium.ch

kundaliniyoga.net

kundaliniyoga.nu

kundaliniyoga.org

naad.net

peacecereal.com

positivemind.com

sacredgems.com

sikhnet.com

SpiritVoyage.com

webreathe.com

yogaguy.com

yogatech.com

yogicnumerology.com

yogitea.com

KUNDALINI YOGA INFORMATION

To find out more about Kundalini Yoga, Yogi Bhajan, 3HO (Healthy, Happy, Holy Organization), and 3HO events such as Summer and Winter Solstice Celebrations, Tantric Courses, Sat Nam Rasayan courses, Teacher-Training Programs, and more, contact:

3HO home page: www.3ho.org
Yogi Bhajan home page:
www.yogibhajan.com
Kundalini Yoga: www.kundaliniyoga.com

To find a Kundalini Yoga center or teacher in your area, contact:
International Kundalini
Yoga Teachers Association (IKYTA)
phone: (505) 753-0423
fax: (505) 753-5982
email: ikyta@newmexico.com
www.kundaliniyoga.com

To receive the latest information about Kundalini Yoga, with yoga sets and meditations, send for "The Science of Keeping Up" Newsletter.
Contact:
3HO International Headquarters
P. O. Box 351149
Los Angeles, CA 90035
phone: (310) 552-3416, fax: (310) 557-8414

SACRED SOURCES

Materials for further study of Kundalini Yoga, meditation, yogic cooking, the yogic healing arts, tantric yoga, as well as music for meditation and relaxation, and all teachings of Yogi Bhajan, can be found through the following sources:

Ancient Healing Ways Catalog

Books, CDs, Tapes, Ayurvedic products, Yogi Teas, Essential Oils, Herbs, and more. Contact for catalog.
P.O. Box 130
Espanola, NM 87532
phone: (800) 359-2940
(outside USA: (505) 747-2860)
Fax: (505) 747-2868
wholesale: (877) 753-5351

Cherdi Kala Music

Audio tapes, CDs, videotapes.
436 North Bedford Drive, Suite 308
Beverly Hills, CA 90210
phone/fax: (310) 838-9989
www.cherdikala.com

Golden Temple Enterprises

Audio and video tapes of Yogi Bhajan's lectures and classes, music tapes and CDs, books. Contact for catalog.
Box 13, Shady Lane
Espanola, NM 87532
phone: (800) 829-3970
fax: (505) 753-5603
GoldenTempleUSA.com

Invincible Recordings
Audio tapes and CDs.
P.O. Box 13054,
Phoenix, AZ 85002
phone: (800) 829-3970
Invinciblemusic.com

Yogi Ji Press
publisher of yogic books
P.O. Box 970
Santa Cruz, NM 87567
phone: (888) 809 0885
fax: (505) 753-9249
email: nam@newmexico.com

For potassium alum orders, contact:
taoskundalini.com

Companion CD for
KUNDALINI YOGA
by Shakta Kaur Khalsa

• This full-length CD contains some of the finest selections of divinely uplifting music from the vast 3HO/Kundalini Yoga repertoire.

• Use with your daily yoga practice, for meditation, deep relaxation, peaceful sleep, or anytime you want to surround yourself with a beautiful sound current!

•Includes a variety of songs and mantras, as well as the sound of the ancient gong.

• Bonus! Includes all mantras used in this book with clear pronunciation, rhythm, and tone.

To hear a selection or to order CD, go to www.SpiritVoyage.com or call toll free 1-888-735-4800

INDEX

ACKNOWLEDGMENTS

Gratitude goes to the following:
My teacher, the master of Kundalini Yoga, Yogi Bhajan, for having
the grace, wisdom, and patience to teach us all these years.
My husband, Kartar Singh Khalsa, and son, Ram Das Singh
Khalsa for their great love and support.

Although the resources for this book came from many KRI
approved sources, the author wishes to acknowledge *Kundalini
Yoga Sadhana Guidelines*, compiled by Gurucharn Singh Khalsa,
Ph.D., *Kundalini Yoga: The Flow of Eternal Power* by Shakti Parwha
Kaur Khalsa, and *Foods for Health and Healing*, by Yogi Bhajan, as
the main sources of reference.

Thanks goes to the following persons for their generous
contributions:
• **Models:** Mary Flinn, Amir Hassan, Gururattan Singh, Kudrat
Kaur Khalsa, Deborah Clapp, Maki Yamamoto, Simran Kaur
Khalsa, Gurubanda Singh Khalsa, Amrit Kaur Khalsa, Siri Sunderi
Kaur Khalsa, Gurukirn Kaur Khalsa, Gurumeet Kaur Khalsa, Sat
Nam Singh Khalsa, Mark (Himat Singh) Dayvault, Gurufathe
Kaur Khalsa, Sat Jivan Kaur Khalsa, Joanne Dugan and Hugo
Moulin, Ella Jones, Ram Das Singh Khalsa, and Madeleine Foster.
• Soho Sanctuary, New York for the use of props.
• Kundalini Yoga East, New York City and Sat Jivan Kaur Khalsa
for use of the gong, and for great advice.
• Everyone at the Kundalini Research Institute (KRI), and most
especially Satya Kaur Khalsa.
• Dr. Dharma Singh Khalsa, Carol Khalsa, Harijot Kaur Khalsa,
Gurucharn Singh Khalsa, and Shakti Parwha Kaur Khalsa for
timely and helpful advice.
• Sat Want Singh Khalsa - Golden Temple photo,
Meditation Chapter

• Jan Carson - three photos of children in Family Yoga section
• Atma Singh Khalsa - two photos of Yogi Bhajan
• Hector Jara (Mukhtiar Singh) - Chakras paintings
• Ravi Tej Singh Khalsa, painting in The King of the Yogis story
• Siri-Kartar Kaur Khalsa, for various paintings of spiritual
masters
• Harimandir Kaur Khalsa for peace prayer painting
Heartfelt thanks goes to all at Dorling Kindersley, and especially
for LaVonne Carlson, Barbara Berger, Mandy Earey, and
Crystal Coble.
Special thanks to Dave King of King Studios for photos.

DK would like to thank Michelle Baxter, Jonathan Bennett,
Nanette Cardon, Megan Clayton, Martin Copeland, Mark Dennis,
Scott Stickland, and Lauren Weiner for their work on this project.
Clothing worn by the models was provided by Capezio
Dance-Theatre Shop, 51st and Broadway, New York City,
(212) 245-2130.

Picture Credits
t = top; b = bottom; l = left; r = right.

Max Alexander: 176bl; Geoff Brightling: 158bl; Jan Carson:
196/197br, tl; Alistiar Duncan: 174; Gables: 178rl Image Bank: 185r;
Hector Jara (Mukhtiar Singh): 37r; 38/39lr; 159r; Harimandir Kaur
Khalsa: 167r; Siri-Kartar Kaur Khalsa: 8tl, 147tl, 155r, 165r; 175tr,
178bl; Atma Singh Khalsa: 9tr, 149tr; Soo Jin Park: 14/15b, 81br;
122l 174bl, 188l; Panoramic Images 180/181br; Tony
Stone: 186b, 187tr, r, br.